0003057329
AF846185
1979

for Dental A...

MEDICAL LIBRARY, CORK REGIONAL HOSPITAL
COLÁISTE NA hOLLSCOILE, CORCAIGH

Níl sé ceaduithe an leabhar seo a choimead thar an dáta is déanaí atá luaite thíos.
This book must be returned not later than the last date stamped below.

24 MAY 1993
09 DEC 1993
23 DEC 1993
03 FEB 1994

WITHDRAWN FROM STOCK

The Library, University College, Cork

M.O. 21,204

24 MAY 1993

Self-Assessment QUESTIONS AND ANSWERS *for Dental Assistants*

Peter L. Erridge

LDS RCS(Eng)

Dental Surgeon, Kent and Canterbury Hospital
Member of the Panel of Examiners for Dental Surgery Assistants

John Wright & Sons Ltd · Bristol 1979

© P. L. Erridge 1979
All Rights Reserved. No part of this publication may be reproduced, stored in a retrieval system, or transmitted, in any form or by any means, electronic, mechanical, photocopying, recording or otherwise, without the prior permission of the Copyright owner.

CIP Data

Erridge, P L
Self assessment questions and answers for dental assistants.
1. Dentistry – Problems, exercises, etc.
2. Dental assistants
I. Title
617.6′0076 RK57

ISBN 0 7236 0524 6

An Leabharlann,
Coláiste na hOllscoile,
Corcaigh

W617·6 ERRI

Printed in England by
BILLING & SONS LTD., GUILDFORD, LONDON AND WORCESTER

Introduction

There are two stages in the learning process; firstly learning the facts, secondly trying to understand these facts and applying them to everyday work. Experience in teaching and in examining Dental Assistants has shown that much time is spent trying to assimilate the facts but not enough effort is expended on their understanding and application.

Therefore it was considered that a book was needed which would encourage the Dental Assistants to question basic facts with the basic questions:- how, what, where, when and why. Furthermore, it is hoped that having been encouraged to have a questioning attitude, the student will maintain and develop this approach to work to the advantage of themselves and to the practice of dentistry.

Some difficulty is always experienced in deciding the level of knowledge and understanding which a D.A. should acquire. The Author hopes that an acceptable compromise has been reached and would be pleased to receive comments from students and teachers.

How to Use This Book

It is suggested that the student reads the relevant section in the textbooks, attends the lecture (if possible) and then reads again the textbook. Only after learning as much as possible about that particular subject should any attempt be made to answer questions in this book, if maximum benefit is to be gained. It is recommended that all the questions on one subject are answered before reference is made to the answer section.

The major part of the book consists of basic questions requiring concise answers. For accuracy of self-marking it is recommended that the answers to each question be written down. In this way differences between what was intended and what was actually expressed will be noted and this should benefit the learning process.

There is a short section in instrument and material layouts for practical procedures. It is important that the lists are written in the order of use as this helps to show understanding of the procedures and to obviate omissions.

Another part is entitled "Short Essay Questions". Each question should be answered with a short essay giving relevant facts in concise sentences. Only when the written answer is as good as it can be should reference be made to the model answers at the back of the book. The model answers contain a skeleton answer together with a marking scheme. The marks give some indication of relative importance of the facts to the answer.

UNIVERSITY COLLEGE Library CORK

The answers to these sections have been kept as concise as possible which will in some cases lead the student to need further information. Reference back to the standard textbooks will clarify most issues. In all cases it is to be hoped that the student will be given maximum support and encouragement by the Dental Surgeon.

The final part contains multiple choice questions. In these questions a statement is made or a question asked. Underneath, several possible answers are given, ONE or MORE of which can be considered the most appropriate answer. This type of question depends upon accuracy of meaning of words both in the question and in the answer. Great care has been taken in devising the questions but it may be that some students will experience problems - the Author hopes these will be few. Note should be made of the answers to a complete section before referring to the answers. This section could be used as final revision.

Acknowledgements

The Author wishes to thank his colleagues who kindly read the manuscript and gave many helpful suggestions; also the Dental Assistants attending the local college course who took part in testing the multiple choice questions.

Particular thanks are due to Mrs J. Atterbury who typed the drafts and the manuscript and to my wife for her advice and forbearance during the preparation of this book.

Table of Contents

Title	Questions Page Numbers	Answers Page Numbers
Oro-Facial Anatomy	1- 2	61- 62
Tooth Anatomy	2- 3	62- 63
Pathology and Microbiology	3- 5	64- 65
Sterilisation	5- 6	65- 66
Preventive Dentistry	6	66- 67
Periodontics	7- 8	67- 69
Caries	8- 9	69- 70
Conservative Dentistry	9- 11	71- 74
Paedodontics	11- 12	74- 75
Crowns and Bridges	12- 13	75- 76
Endodontics	13- 15	76- 79
Physiology	15- 17	79- 81
First Aid	17- 18	81- 83
Drugs	18	83- 84
Local Anaesthesia	18- 20	84- 86
Extractions and Minor Oral Surgery	20- 22	86- 89
General Disease	22- 23	89- 90
Radiography	23- 25	90- 93
Orthodontics	25- 26	93- 94
General Anaesthesia	26- 28	94- 97
Materials	28- 29	98- 99
Prosthetics	29- 31	99-102
Instrument and Material Layouts	31	102-104
Short Essay		
Pathology, Microbiology and Sterilisation	32	104-105
Anatomy and Physiology	32	105-106
Instruments, Materials and Drugs	32	106-108
Dental Disease	33	108-109
Restorative Dentistry	33	109-110

Short Essay (Continued)		
Anaesthesia, First Aid and Minor Oral Surgery	33- 34	110-112
Multiple Choice		
General	34- 36	113
Oral Anatomy	36- 40	113
Microbiology	40- 41	113
Materials	41- 42	113
Prosthetics	43- 45	114
Radiography	45- 48	114
Anaesthesia	48- 52	114
Caries	52- 53	115
Children's Dentistry	54- 56	115
Conservation	56- 60	115

PART 1
QUESTIONS

Oro-Facial Anatomy

1. Which bones form the majority of the upper jaw?
2. Which bony cavity is part of the upper jaw?
3. Which part of the upper jaw forms the floor of the nose?
4. Occasionally the roof of the mouth does not develop properly in a baby. What is this abnormality called?
5. Where in the mouth is the tuberosity found?
6. What is a foramen?
7. What is the alveolar bone?
8. What is the alveolar ridge?
9. The ascending ramus of the mandible has two prominent parts. What are they called? What is their function?
10. What is the name of the opening in the bone on the inner surface of the mandible, and what is its function?
11. Where is the mental foramen to be found in the dentate adult?
12. How can you recognise a dislocated jaw?
13. Healthy gingivae are pinker than the remainder of the mucous membrane of the mouth. Why is this?
14. a) Name the ridges of tissue in the roof of the mouth.
    b) Of what are they composed?
15. What is the function of the soft palate?
16. Where is the buccal sulcus found?
17. What is the name applied to the soft tissue lining the oral cavity?
18. What are the main functions of the tongue?
19. Where are the salivary glands situated?
20. What are the main functions of saliva?
21. What causes the increase or decrease in the flow of saliva?
22. Swelling of the parotid gland is usually associated with which condition?

23. Which muscles are mainly concerned with the closure of the jaws?

24. Which muscle is mainly concerned with helping to swing the mandible to either side?

25. Which muscles control lip movements?

26. Why is the mylohyoid muscle important in denture construction?

27. Which nerve supplies the muscles of mastication?

28. Which cranial nerve supplies the teeth and jaws, and what are its three main branches?

29. Sensory nerves of the lower lip are part of which nerve?

30. Why does the tongue usually go numb when an inferior dental nerve block is given?

31. To extract a lower permanent second molar under local anaesthesia, the Dental Surgeon will give the patient which injections and why?

32. How does the density of bone in the area of the mandibular permanent molars affect the local anaesthesia technique used by Dental Surgeons?

33. Give the names of the branches of the maxillary nerve, of dental interest.

34. When the jaw moves from open to closed; what muscle actions take place?

35. Bone is covered by a fibrous membrane, what is this tissue called?

<u>Tooth Anatomy</u>

1. Which surface of a tooth touches:
   a) the lips
   b) the lower surface of the side of the tongue
   c) the upper surface of the side of the tongue
   d) the cheek
   e) the tooth in front
   f) the tooth behind.

2. What is a tooth germ?

3. At what age do the deciduous teeth normally start to erupt?

4. Visually, how do deciduous teeth differ from permanent teeth?

5. Which permanent tooth, or teeth, commonly has, or have:
   a) no cusps
   b) one cusp
   c) four cusps
   d) five cusps
   e) the cusps of Carabelli
   f) a conical root
   g) a flattened root
   h) two roots
   i) three roots
   j) four roots.

6. Why do deciduous molar teeth have divergent roots?

7. Which vitamins help in the formation of teeth?

8. Which type of teeth have no deciduous predecessors?

9. Which tissues constitute the crown of a tooth?

10. Which tissues constitute the root of a tooth?

11. How is a tooth held in its socket?

12. Where is the inter-radicular bone found?

13. Where is the apical foramen usually found?

14. What is an odontoblast?

15. Where is enamel thicker?

16. What is the name given to the area where the enamel and dentine join?

17. What is the microscopic structure of enamel?

18. How is pain conducted through dentine?

19. Which dental tissue contains millions of fibres, and what is their function?

20. Is cementum sensitive?

21. How does the size of the pulp of a permanent tooth alter during life?

22. The tooth pulp contains several types of tissue. Give their names.

23. What is a dental contact point?

24. Which is usually the first permanent tooth to erupt and at about what age?

Pathology and Microbiology

1. What is the approximate size of a) bacteria, b) viruses?

2. How may infection be spread?

3. What are the ideal living conditions for most micro-organisms?

4. Where, about the body, are micro-organisms most commonly found?

5. How may micro-organisms enter the body?

6. A person may carry a disease organism without having the disease him or herself. What name is applied to such a person?

7. What are the factors which decide whether a harmful infection occurs?

8. What is the name of the condition in which micro-organisms are present in the bloodstream without clinical symptoms?

9. What is meant by immunity?

10. What is the cause of lockjaw?

11. Denture sore mouth is associated with which group of micro-organisms?

12. Briefly define
    a) disinfectants
    b) antiseptics
    c) antibiotics.

13. Why should handpieces and the spray nozzle be wiped with an antiseptic, or sterilised, between patients?

14. Which term is applied when micro-organisms are present in the blood and body tissues with clinical symptoms?

15. What is pus and what does it contain?

16. What is a collection of pus called?

17. The mouth is full of micro-organisms. Why do not all tooth sockets become infected?

18. In dentistry particular care is taken against spreading which blood-borne liver disease?

19. Why might a patient produce a chronic inflammatory reaction rather than an acute inflammatory reaction?

20. What are the principles in the treatment of infection?

21. What are the possible outcomes of acute inflammation?

22. Why do plasma and white cells pass into tissues in acute inflammation?

23. What is a chronic inflammatory reaction?

24. What is a cyst?

25. What is meant by the term 'necrosis'?

26. What is a tumour?

27. Give the names of the two main types of tumour. Briefly state their main differences.

28. What is meant by
    a) hypertrophy
    b) hyperplasia
    c) atrophy.

Sterilisation

1. What should a D.A. do with used dental instruments when the patient leaves the surgery?

2. What are three disadvantages of chemical solutions for sterilising?

3. How are cheatle forceps sterilised?

4. Why should instruments be rendered physically clean before sterilisation?

5. How should instruments which have been in contact with a patient's blood be sterilised?

6. Which sterilisation methods can spoil the temper of metal instruments?

7. Name two commercial methods of sterilising disposable items?

8. How is it possible to kill spores using boiling water?

9. Why is flaming not a suitable method for sterilising metal instruments?

10. Why should the door of an autoclave not be opened during sterilisation?

11. After sterilisation, instruments removed from the steriliser can easily become unsterile. How may this be prevented?

UNIVERSITY COLLEGE CORK Library

12. Why should used disposable needles and scapel blades be handled very carefully?

13. Why should syringes and needles be broken before disposal?

Preventive Dentistry

1. What five local factors can lead to gingival inflammation?

2. What are the main factors associated with dental caries?

3. How are teeth naturally cleaned?

4. Name the four constituents of plaque apart from water.

5. What harmful substances are formed by plaque?

6. Why is it important for an expectant mother to have adequate calcium and vitamins in her diet?

7. How does fluoride toothpaste help to prevent caries?

8. How may fluoride be taken by a child to be incorporated into a forming tooth?

9. What is the effect on teeth of taking too many fluoride tablets for a prolonged period of time?

10. What factors assist normal formation of bones and teeth?

11. What are the benefits of mouth brushing?

12. What are the important factors in selecting a new toothbrush?

13. How may patients clean their teeth apart from the use of a toothbrush?

14. Toothpastes contain certain amounts of detergent and abrasive material and are alkaline. What is the purpose of each constituent?

15. Why is it important to clean the teeth properly after the last food and drink at night?

16. How can a patient be shown areas of the mouth which are not being cleaned properly?

17. What tooth brushing advice is usually given by the Dental Surgeon to patients whose gums bleed?

18. In what three ways can the Dental Surgeon reduce the incidence of fissure caries?

Periodontics

1. How deep is a normal gingival pocket?
2. Why are the gingivae in gingivitis redder than usual?
3. What is periodontitis?
4. How can patients help to prevent periodontal disease?
5. Where and how does periodontal disease usually start?
6. Give three of the consequences of having an unopposed tooth.
7. What can be the consequences on the surrounding teeth of the loss of one tooth?
8. Which tissues are concerned in periodontal disease?
9. What is calculus?
10. Name the two types of calculus.
11. Faulty tooth brushing can damage which three tissues?
12. Why do many Dental Surgeons recommend brushing "the way the tooth grows"?
13. When does breathing affect the gums harmfully?
14. How does diet help to maintain healthy gums?
15. Give examples of drugs and chemicals which have harmful effects on the gingivae.
16. In which particular areas is supra-gingival calculus commonly found?
17. Why is it found there?
18. What is the importance of saliva in the formation of calculus?
19. Why is calculus in a periodontal pocket dark in colour?
20. Why does subgingival calculus collect progressively in an apical direction?
21. Acute ulcerative gingivitis leads to damage of which particular area of gum tissue?
22. Give at least four of the important features of acute ulcerative gingivitis.

23. What three measures does the Dental Surgeon ask the patient to carry out in acute ulcerative gingivitis?

24. When is surgery to periodontal tissues carried out rather than a gingivectomy?

25. What are the constituents of a periodontal pack?

26. What is a periodontal abscess?

27. How does a periodontal abscess develop?

<u>Caries</u>

1. Briefly define caries.

2. Where are the common sites for dental caries to occur in the mouth, and why does it favour these sites?

3. Give three ways in which the Dental Surgeon may detect dental caries.

4. Which are the most common places to find plaque?

5. Why is plaque less common on palatal surfaces of teeth?

6. Why is plaque an important factor in the caries process?

7. What is the effect of saliva on dental caries incidence?

8. How is the initial lesion in enamel caries of a smooth surface recognised?

9. How does the Dental Surgeon produce a similar effect during one form of dental treatment?

10. How is the decay process aided by the early caries lesion?

11. Why is it that an apparently small cavity in a tooth can turn out to be so large?

12. When a cavity just involves dentine, patients often complain of pain with hot drinks and hot food. Why is this?

13. How can the tooth itself delay the caries process from reaching the pulp?

14. Why does an inflamed pulp cause pain?

15. In general terms give two main causes of pulp death.

16. What may happen to an untreated periapical abscess?

17. What is a "gumboil"?

18. Dental caries is relatively uncommon in lower permanent incisor teeth. Why is this?

19. What is the effect on the teeth, and the incidence of dental decay in children, of one part per million of fluoride in water?

20. Define the words attrition, abrasion and erosion.

Conservative Dentistry

1. What are four reasons for filling a tooth?

2. Give two factors which influence a Dental Surgeon's choice of filling materials.

3. Why is the high speed drill usually used to remove enamel?

4. What is meant by the process of micro-leakage of dental restorations?

5. Why are conventional steel burs not used at very high speed?

6. What factors does a Dental Surgeon consider when shaping a tooth cavity?

7. How may a tooth cavity be kept free from saliva?

8. Why are matrix bands and strips fitted to teeth?

9. Why are temporary fillings used?

10. Why are calcium hydroxide materials used in deep cavities?

11. Give reasons for the use of cavity linings.

12. Give three methods of mixing amalgam.

13. What are the results of excess mercury in an amalgam restoration?

14. How may amalgam become contaminated by moisture?

15. What will be the result of moisture contamination of amalgam?

16. Why should amalgam be used immediately after mixing?

17. What are the effects to the D.A. of the handling of amalgam?

18. What are the reasons for carving an amalgam filling?

19. Why does the Dental Surgeon condense the amalgam into the cavity?

20. How long is it before a patient may apply pressure to a recently inserted amalgam filling?

21. After an amalgam filling has fully set, how may it be "finished"?

22. What are the reasons for polishing fillings?

23. What is the difference between a cutting and a finishing bur?

24. Why is amalgam commonly used to fill cavities in posterior teeth?

25. Why should waste amalgam be stored under water?

26. Why should amalgam not be handled?

27. What are the uses of zinc oxide - eugenol cement?

28. How and why does an amalgam cavity differ from a gold inlay cavity?

29. Why might a gold inlay be used instead of amalgam to restore a tooth?

30. Briefly, what is the main difference between the direct and indirect inlay impression techniques in the laboratory?

31. Which materials are commonly used to obtain an indirect impression of an inlay cavity?

32. Why is an astringent cord sometimes used before any indirect impression is taken?

33. When fitting a gold inlay what does the Dental Surgeon check?

34. Why are the margins of a gold restoration "burnished"?

35. Which materials are used to cement crowns and inlays?

36. How should cements be mixed for cementing crowns?

37. Why is a rubber dam used when inserting fillings?

38. Which materials used for dental restorations are not mixed by the D.A?

39. Briefly, how is silicate filling powder made?

40. What are the main constituents of silicate cement liquid?

41. Why should the cap of the bottle of the liquid part of silicate cement be replaced immediately after use?

42. What may cause grey discolouration of silicate cement?

43. What is the ideal mixing temperature of silicate cement?

44. What are the disadvantages of silicate cements?

45. Why should silicate fillings be coated with petroleum jelly or varnish?

46. What is the effect of saliva contamination on silicate cements during setting?

47. Why do silicate and composite fillings need a lining?

48. What are Agate, Stellite and bone spatulas used for and why?

49. What are the advantages of composites over other filling materials?

50. In simple terms what are the constituents of composite filling materials?

51. How can the setting time of "two paste" composites be retarded?

52. a) What are the main uses of glass ionomer cements?
    b) What is their particularly useful property ?

53. What precautions can a patient take to reduce the chance of traumatic damage to incisor teeth when playing contact sports?

<u>Paedodontics</u>

1. What are the most important aspects of dentistry for a two and a half year old child?

2. What advice can be given about teeth to parents of young children?

3. When do the following teeth usually
   a) Start to calcify
   b) Start to erupt
      1) Deciduous central incisor
      2) Permanent central incisor
      3) Permanent first molar
      4) First premolar.

4. How does enamel and dentine of deciduous teeth differ from these tissues in permanent teeth?

5. For what reasons does the Dental Surgeon try to conserve deciduous molar teeth?

6. Why is it difficult to obtain a good apical seal when root filling the permanent upper central incisor of a six and a half year old child?

7. What is meant by pulp mummification?

8. Why is it not usually possible to root fill completely a deciduous molar tooth?

9. In an injury of a permanent incisor involving exposure of some dentine, why does the Dental Surgeon cover the tooth with a temporary crown?

10. Why do some traumatised anterior teeth discolour?

11. What is meant by vital pulpotomy?

12. What tests would the Dental Surgeon apply to traumatised permanent anterior teeth and why would these tests be used?

13. How can deciduous teeth lead to malocclusion in the permanent dentition?

14. What are the reasons for carrying out orthodontic treatment?

<u>Crowns and Bridges</u>

1. Define what is meant by a crown restoration.

2. What conservative treatment is likely to be carried out on an anterior tooth in which almost all of the crown has been lost?

3. Why is it usually necessary to remove at least 2mm of tooth substance when preparing a crown?

4. Which materials are used to take the detailed impression of a crown or bridge preparation?

5. What type of scissors should be used for trimming copper and aluminium rings?

6. Apart from the detailed impression of the crown preparation what other information does the dental technician require before making a crown?

7. Why is astringent cord used before taking crown impressions?

8. What might a "high spot" on a crown lead to?

9. Give three reasons why temporary crowns are fitted between impressions and fit appointments.

10. a) What is a bridge? b) Name the parts of a bridge.

11. Bridges are usually constructed of which materials?

12. What factors are considered before a dental bridge is designed?

13. What are the advantages of bridges over partial dentures?

14. What materials are used to fix a bridge to supporting teeth?

15. Why should these materials have a runny consistency when used?

<u>Endodontics</u>

1. What is meant by the word 'endodontics'?

2. What are the basic objectives of root canal therapy?

3. Why are radiographs taken before commencing root canal therapy?

4. How many root canals are usually found in:
   a) upper lateral incisor d) lower lateral incisor
   b) upper first premolar e) lower first premolar
   c) upper first molar f) lower first permanent molar.

5. What are the main causes of pulpitis?

6. How can the pulp of an infected tooth sometimes still be vital?

7. What is the commonest cause of a periapical abscess?

8. Why is a tooth with a periapical abscess tender?

9. How are the following sterilised in the surgery
   a) paper points b) gutta percha points.

10. What is the ideal method of sterilising root canal instruments?

11. Which two classes of drugs are used to "sterilise" a root canal?

12. Why are chemicals such as hydrogen peroxide and sodium hypochlorite used in root canal therapy?

13. When should a safety chain be attached to root canal instruments?

14. What are the five important stages in root canal therapy?

15. Give reasons why a rubber dam is used in endodontics.

16. How may a root canal be kept dry and free from contamination if a rubber dam cannot be used?

17. What are smooth broaches used for in endodontics?

18. List the types of root canal reamer.

19. What are the uses of:
a) reamers
b) root canal files
c) rotary paste fillers.

20. Why should a root canal be shaped carefully?

21. What is the action of a Giromatic handpiece?

22. What are two advantages of Giromatic reamers?

23. Give two disadvantages of Giromatic reamers.

24. What are the uses of paper points in endodontics?

25. Why are intermediate root dressings inserted?

26. Can a tooth root have more than one apical opening?

27. Is the apical foramen always at the apex of a root?

28. How can a Dental Surgeon judge that the gutta percha or silver point will reach the root apex?

29. Why is a root sealing paste used as part of the root filling?

30. Why are gutta percha points or silver points usually used when root filling a tooth?

31. Why, in many cases, is only the apical third of the root canal filled?

32. In which cases might a Dental Surgeon prefer to use a silver point?

33. Give two ways in which a periapical abscess may be drained.

34. What instructions are given to a patient about mouth care after drainage of an abscess?

35. For what reasons would a Dental Surgeon extirpate a vital pulp?

36. What is an apicectomy?

37. What is meant by a retrograde amalgam?

Physiology

1. What is physiology?

2. What is required before energy can be released in the body?

3. What is this energy used for?

4. What are the main excretory organs of the body?

5. Define the two types of respiration which take place in the body.

6. Name, in order, the passages and tissues through which oxygen passes from the environment to a pulmonary capillary.

7. What are the basic principles of all types of artificial respiration?

8. What are the common causes of rapid breathing in a healthy person?

9. How is oxygen transported in the blood?

10. How is carbon dioxide transported in the blood?

11. What are the main parts of the blood circulation system? (Use a correct order of circulation).

12. What is meant by "the pulse"?

13. What are the names of the chambers of the heart? What is the function of each?

14. What is the function of heart valves?

15. Which type of blood is found in the pulmonary vein?

16. How do the heart muscles obtain their blood?

17. What are the main constituents of a blood clot?

18. What is the purpose of the blood clotting process?

UNIVERSITY COLLEGE Library CORK

19. What is the role of blood platelets in blood coagulation?

20. What is the volume of blood in the average adult?

21. How much blood is ejected from each ventricle at each heart beat in an average adult in the resting state?

22. What is anaemia?

23. What are the main constituents of blood and their proportions?

24. What is the function of white blood cells?

25. What is the function of lymph glands?

26. What is the function of the lymphatic system?

27. Why is digestion necessary?

28. What are the essential constituents of the diet?

29. Where does the first stage of digestion take place?

30. Briefly explain what happens in the first stage of digestion.

31. What protective actions occur during swallowing?

32. What is the action of the tongue in mastication?

33. What is the purpose of the masticatory process?

34. What is meant by a digestive enzyme?

35. "The diet should be adequate and balanced". What is meant by this statement?

36. Give the important factors which affect the amount of food required by a person.

37. How long may the gastric digestive process take?

38. Why does the alimentary canal secrete mucous?

39. Why is gastric juice acid?

40. Give two examples of foods which are absorbed through the stomach walls into the blood stream.

41. What part of the digestive process takes place
a) in the ileum
b) in the colon.

42. Why are nasal and oral secretions necessary to perceive the senses of smell and taste?

43. Where are the majority of taste buds to be found?

44. What are the functions of the epithelial tissues?

45. What are the functions of the skeleton?

46. Which cells are responsible for remodelling bone?

First Aid

1. Why is it important for a Dental Surgeon to get a full medical history, and to know of any drugs which the patient is taking?

2. In which areas can a D.A. help to prevent accidents to patients and staff in the practice?

3. How can a D.A. help to prevent injury to a conscious patient during dental treatment?

4. List some common causes of collapse.

5. What is shock?

6. What are the symptoms of shock?

7. What are the signs of shock?

8. What are the causes of shock?

9. How would you treat a patient with shock?

10. What are the consequences of severe haemorrhage?

11. What is the first aid treatment of non-dental haemorrhage?

12. A patient collapses on the floor and is having convulsions. What might be the reasons for these convulsions?

13. What is the difference between a burn and a scald?

14. What is the first aid treatment of burns?

15. Give the first aid treatment in cases of electrocution.

16. Give the signs of an epileptic fit - grand mal.

17. How should you help a patient having an epileptic fit?

18. What are the signs and symptoms of fainting?

19. Why might a pregnant woman faint even in the horizontal position in a dental chair?

20. What first aid treatment would you give to a person with a suspected fractured bone?

Drugs

1. What is the use of the following drugs
   a) an analgesic
   b) a hypnotic
   c) a tranquilliser
   d) a sedative.

2. What advice should be given to a patient regarding aspirin tablets?

3. What are the differences between an antiseptic and an antibiotic?

4. Drugs are sometimes given to prevent disease. What is the term used to describe this type of therapy?

5. Why might a patient be taking anti-coagulant drugs?

6. What problems can arise in penicillin therapy?

7. In which medical condition might penicillin be given prophylactically prior to dental treatment?

8. Why is premedication sometimes given to a patient?

9. How is premedication administered in dentistry? Name one drug used.

10. Why might a patient be taking steroid drugs?

11. What is the effect of steroid drugs on the body?

12. A patient might state that because of a drug prescribed by the doctor he is not to eat cheese, yeast extracts, etc. Why should this be reported to the Dental Surgeon?

13. What are the basic principles in treatment of poisoning?

14. What is a fungicide? Give an example of a fungicide used in dentistry.

15. What is a mummifying agent?

Local Anaesthesia

1. Give three reasons for the use of local anaesthesia in dentistry.

2. In which three basic ways can local anaesthesia be obtained?

3. What is an intra-osseus injection?

4. How does a local anaesthetic drug work?

5. Why is a local anaesthetic solution seldom used where there is an infection?

6. What are the uses of a surface anaesthetic?

7. How can the needle diaphragm of the local anaesthetic cartridge be disinfected?

8. What are the contents of any local anaesthetic cartridge?

9. What are the advantages of disposable needles for local anaesthesia?

10. Why should local anaesthetic solution be at about body temperature when it is injected?

11. What should a D.A. do before handing an unguarded local anaesthetic syringe to the Dental Surgeon?

12. Why should patients be offered a mouth wash immediately after receiving a local anaesthetic injection?

13. What types of disposable needles are there?

14. Which nerves are affected by a mandibular nerve block?

15. Why do most local anaesthetics contain a vaso-constrictor?

16. What is the advantage of the aspirating syringe for the administration of local anaesthetic solutions?

17. What might be the consequences of injecting local anaesthetic solution into a blood vessel?

18. What is the most common complication associated with the giving of local anaesthetics, and what is the usual cause?

19. How may a local anaesthetic syringe needle cause complications when a local anaesthetic is administered?

20. Why should the same local anaesthetic cartridge not be used on more than one patient?

21. What is paraesthesia?

22. What are the causes of paraesthesia?

23. Why might a patient experience difficulty in opening the mouth (trismus), following a local anaesthetic injection?

Extractions and Minor Oral Surgery

1. What are the two main reasons for extracting teeth?

2. How many roots do the following teeth commonly possess:
   a) lower deciduous molars
   b) upper deciduous molars
   c) incisors
   d) lower premolars
   e) upper first premolars
   f) upper first permanent molars
   g) lower second permanent molars.

3. Give simple patient instructions to reduce haemorrhage following tooth extraction.

4. How does a tooth socket heal normally?

5. What is a "dry socket"?

6. How does a "dry socket" heal?

7. What is the use of a periosteal elevator?

8. What instrument might the Dental Surgeon use to hold soft tissues when suturing?

9. Why are patients advised not to rinse, and to avoid raising their blood pressure for 24 hours after dental extractions?

10. Why are hot salt water mouth washes advised, starting 24 hours after an extraction?

11. What instruments should be laid out for suturing?

12. What materials are used in dental suturing?

13. Why are non-resorbable sutures usually removed after 5 to 7 days?

14. What are cheatle forceps used for?

15. How can the D.A. help to allay a patient's fears?

16. What is meant by minor oral surgery?

17. List some examples of minor oral surgery procedures.

18. What is an apicectomy?

19. What is a biopsy?

20. What should you do with tissue for biopsy?

21. What are the uses of:
    a) retractors
    b) Warrick James' elevators
    c) Cryer's elevators.

22. What is meant by an impacted tooth?

23. Name four types of wisdom tooth impaction.

24. What pathological conditions may be associated with a partially erupted impacted tooth?

25. What factors help a Dental Surgeon to decide the line of a surgical incision?

26. What is the reason for using curved cutting suture needles in the mouth?

27. Why is strict sterility necessary in minor oral surgery procedures?

28. What is osteomyelitis?

29. When carrying out surgical extractions of lower wisdom teeth, the Dental Surgeon and his assistant must take care not to damage a nerve lying close to the inner surface of the mandible. What is this nerve called?

30. What is an oro-antral fistula?

31. How might an oro-antral fistula be caused during dental treatment?

32. What instructions are given to a patient to help to prevent an oro-antral fistula?

33. What is an abscess sinus?

34. What is the commonest cause of a dental abscess in young people?

35. What is an alveolectomy, and what are common reasons for its use?

36. What is meant by pericoronitis?

37. Why does pericoronitis occur?

38. Why do surgeons and their assistants wear head caps and face masks when operating?

39. Name instruments which may be used to remove bone in dentistry.

40. What is the use of a Hunt's syringe?

41. Why are disposable scalpel blades used for surgery, nowadays?

42. What are the uses of Coupland's chisels?

43. What is blood clotting?

44. When does primary haemorrhage occur?

45. When does reactionary haemorrhage occur?

46. Why does reactionary haemorrhage occur?

47. What could a D.A. do to help a patient who returns with a bleeding socket?

48. When does secondary haemorrhage occur?

49. What is the usual cause of secondary haemorrhage?

<u>General Disease</u>

1. What is the term applied to the body's reaction to irritation?

2. What is the difference between the symptoms and the signs of disease?

3. What is a non pathenogenic organism?

4. What factors help to decide whether a pathenogenic organism actually causes disease?

5. How may infection spread in the body?

6. What is an abscess and what are its contents?

7. What is meant by the term "fever"?

8. There are two types of inflammation. What are they called? How do they differ?

9. What is an ulcer?

10. Why are antibiotics given before dental surgery to patients who have had rheumatic heart disease?

11. What is a haemophiliac?

12. What is a haemorrhage?

13. What is the physiological arrest of haemorrhage called?

14. What is a thrombus?

15. What damage can a thrombus cause?

16. What is meant by the term "a stroke"?

17. Why are some patients with cardiovascular disease sometimes given anticoagulant drugs?

18. In patients with cardiovascular disease, or on anti-coagulant drugs, how might their dental treatment be altered?

19. What is bronchitis?

20. What are the common causes of chronic bronchitis?

21. What are the signs of chronic bronchitis which a D.A. might notice?

22. What is Bell's Palsy?

23. What is "diabetes"?

24. How is "diabetes" important to the Dental Surgeon?

25. Name the vitamin whose
    a) presence maintains healthy mucous membranes
    b) total lack leads to blindness
    c) lack leads to scurvy
    d) lack leads to rickets
    e) lack may cause soreness at the corners of the mouth.

Radiography

1. Why must care be taken with the use of X-rays?

2. What is the effect of X-rays on an X-ray film?

3. Why do metal fillings appear white on radiographs?

4. What is X radiation?

5. What is a radiograph?

6. What precautions must be taken when storing X-ray films?

7. How are extra-oral films prepared for use?

8. What four factors affect the exposure time of intra-oral films?

9. What can a Dental Surgeon learn from a bite wing radiograph?

10. What is used to keep the exposure time of extra-oral films to a minimum?

11. What is the main use of a dental periapical X-ray film?

12. Which teeth are usually visible on an oblique lateral radiograph?

13. What hard structures are shown on an orthopantomograph?

14. Which tissues of the body are particularly sensitive to X-radiation (6 examples)?

15. How may a D.A. avoid excessive radiation when films are being taken?

16. What general precautions can be taken to prevent excessive radiation?

17. How may excessive radiation be detected?

18. How can a D.A. test the efficiency of a dark room?

19. Why can X-ray films be opened "safely" under a safelight?

20. What does the emulsion on the surface of an X-ray film consist of?

21. What particular care must a D.A. take when opening a film packet?

22. Before starting the developing process for a batch of radiographs, what procedures must a D.A. observe?

23. Why should the film be agitated in the developer?

24. Why should spots of developer or fixer be washed off the skin or clothes immediately?

25. Why is it necessary for a film to stay in the developer and fixer for an accurately measured length of time?

26. Why are films washed in running water following their removal from the developer?

27. Give four reasons why exposed films are placed in a fixing solution.

28. Give two causes of:
a) faint images on radiographs b) film fogging.

29. What are the reasons for a radiograph having only a partial image?

30. Why should radiographs be dried before filing away?

31. How should dental radiographs be stored?

Orthodontics

1. What is the meaning of the word "orthodontics"?

2. What does the orthodontist study?

3. What is the main purpose of orthodontics?

4. What is meant by malocclusion?

5. What are some causes of malocclusion?

6. What is meant in orthodontics by:
a) overjet
b) overbite
c) overcrowding.

7. Briefly, what is meant by a Class I, II and III incisor relationship?

8. What are the three most essential items which the D.A. should put out for orthodontic diagnosis and treatment planning, before the patient is called to the surgery?

9. How is it possible that teeth can be moved in bone by means of orthodontic appliances?

10. Why does the orthodontist usually prefer to extract upper first premolars in Class II cases?

11. What is the name given to the fold of tissue joining the upper lip to the gum in the midline?

12. Why might an Orthodontist want this tissue removed, and what is the operation called?

13. What is meant by a fixed orthodontic appliance?

14. What are the advantages of removable appliances?

15. What are the disadvantages of removable appliances?

16. What is a crib, a labial bow and a spring?

17. What instructions should be given to a patient when a removable appliance is fitted?

General Anaesthesia

1. What is general anaesthesia?

2. How is general anaesthesia produced?

3. What are the indications for giving a general anaesthetic?

4. Which general anaesthetic drugs are administered by:
a) inhalation b) injection
for dental anaesthesia?

5. Why should the drugs in the emergency kit be checked regularly?

6. What sterilized equipment should be laid out ready for a dental general anaesthetic?

7. Why should the name of the patient's current medical practitioner be written on a patient's record card?

8. How often should a patient's medical history and drug record be checked?

9. Why should the patient be accompanied by a D.A. throughout a general anaesthetic?

10. What is endotracheal anaesthesia?

11. What are the most important advantages of endotracheal anaesthesia?

12. How do gaseous anaesthetics get to the brain?

13. What are the advantages and disadvantages of administering general anaesthetics via an intravenous route?

14. What are the characteristics of nitrous oxide?

15. What is the usual minimum percentage of oxygen administered with nitrous oxide, and why is it necessary?

16. What does the word "hypoxia" mean?

17. How can severe hypoxia be detected?

18. How is halothane administered?

19. Why is halothane used with nitrous oxide and oxygen?

20. How is methohexitone administered?

21. How should an anaesthetic machine be set up for a general anaesthetic?

22. How can a patient's fears of dentistry be allayed?

23. What are the duties of a D.A. when receiving a patient who is about to have a general anaesthetic?

24. How can the D.A. reassure the patient before a general anaesthetic?

25. Why should patients be asked not to eat or drink for at least 4 hours before a dental general anaesthetic?

26. What could be the results of failure to observe this advice?

27. What is the effect of a foreign body's touching the vocal cords of an anaesthetised patient?

28. If an anaesthetised patient makes a crowing noise, why is this, and what is the condition called?

29. Why are throat packs used during general anaesthesia?

30. Why is it important not to talk whilst a general anaesthetic is being given to a patient?

31. Why do many Anaesthetists insist on giving dental general anaesthetics to patients who are in a supine position?

32. How should a patient recovering from a general anaesthetic be "monitored"?

33. Into which position should a patient be placed during recovery from a general anaesthetic?

34. What are the commonest causes of patient collapse associated with dental general anaesthesia? Place in order of frequency of occurrence.

35. Why should patients not use machinery for at least 12 hours after a general anaesthetic or intravenous sedation?

36. What is meant by sedation techniques in dentistry?

37. What are the advantages of intravenous premedication?

38. What are the post operative instructions, for the recovery period, when conservation only, will be performed with a sedation technique?

39. What actions should be taken when a patient collapses?

40. How can the dental team ensure that a collapsed patient gets plenty of oxygen?

41. When a patient loses consciousness why is it important to ensure a good oxygen intake?

42. When a person faints there has been inadequate oxygenated blood flow to the brain. Where is the blood to be found?

43. A person who faints will naturally fall to the ground. How does this aid recovery?

44. What is the first aid treatment of cardiac arrest?

Materials

1. What are the uses of zinc oxide in dentistry?

2. What are the uses of dental cements in dentistry?

3. A permanent filling material expands and contracts with temperature changes. Why is this necessary?

4. Give examples of the forms in which wax is supplied for dental use.

5. Two types of material can be used to obtain an accurate fit to edges of special trays. What are they?

6. What are the usual errors in mixing alginate impression material?

7. Which materials are used for gold inlay impressions?

8. Give three uses for thermoplastic impression materials.

9. How is impression composition prepared for use for full mouth impressions?

10. When preparing thermoplastic materials, what happens if they are made much too hot?

11. What are the dental uses of gutta percha?

12. In what procedures is articulating paper used?

13. What are the ideal requirements of a temporary filling?

14. Which materials are used for temporary crowns?

15. Which materials can be used as fissure sealants?

16. How do acid etch materials bond to the enamel?

Prosthetics

1. Give some examples of non-dental prostheses.

2. What are the three main reasons for patients requiring full dentures?

3. What is a partial denture?

4. Name the materials which are commonly used as bases for partial dentures.

5. What impression materials may be used to obtain impressions of an edentulous mouth?

6. a) What complication can occur with a patient when taking impressions, and,
   b) Why?

7. Give three methods by which alginate can be retained in an impression tray.

8. Why is it important that an impression does not become detached?

9. An alginate impression ideally should be cast within 20 minutes. Why is this?

10. What is a functional impression?

11. What should a D.A. do with an alginate impression after the Dental Surgeon has removed it from the mouth?

12. What will happen if an alginate impression is allowed to get too dry or too wet and what will be the consequences?

13. What should be the temperature of the materials used for mixing alginates?

14. Why is a special tray impression sometimes taken?

15. How does the Dental Surgeon obtain the greatest accuracy of the flange edges of an impression?

16. When taking the so-called 'bite' what will the Dental Surgeon wish to show the Dental Technician?

17. What needs to be recorded at the 'bite' stage apart from the 'bite'?

18. Why is there a try-in stage in full denture construction?

19. What does the Dental Surgeon check at the try-in?

20. What would be the appearance of patients with dentures having:
    a) too great a vertical dimension
    b) too little denture support?

21. How may a Dental Surgeon and his Technician make denture teeth look more natural?

22. Why is the posterior edge of an upper denture made to press more firmly into the mucosa than the remainder of the fitting surface?

23. How should dentures be stored when not in the mouth and why is this?

24. Why might articulating paper be used at the 'fit' appointment?

25. What advice will be given to a patient when new dentures are fitted?

26. Why do many patients find some difficulty in controlling a lower full denture?

27. What is a soft lining?

28. How may the fit of a full denture be restored?

29. What is the name applied to the overgrowth of soft tissue associated with a denture flange which is cutting into a patient's mouth?

30. What materials are commonly used to obtain a reline impression?

31. What is a tissue conditioner?

32. What is meant by an immediate denture?

33. What is the major disadvantage of immediate dentures?

34. List the advantages of immediate dentures.

35. Why should extracted posterior teeth be replaced with a partial denture?

36. What is a skeleton denture?

37. What is a lingual bar?

38. There are three basic types of design for partial dentures. What are they?

39. What particular things are being looked for by the Dental Surgeon when he examines the mouth prior to making new full dentures?

40. How can the cleanliness, or otherwise, of dentures be demonstrated to patients?

41. Why are suction pads not fitted to upper dentures any longer?

42. a) What is the post-dam line?
    b) What is its function?

Instrument and Material Layouts

List in order of use the instruments and materials needed for each of the following procedures.

1. Administering a local anaesthetic by injection.

2. Simple extraction of upper second premolar under local anaesthesia.

3. Repair of oral mucosa by suturing.

4. Removal of lower first permanent molar roots.

5. Biopsy of soft tissue.

6. First visit for septic root canal therapy.

7. Taking impressions for a porcelain jacket crown, after the preparation stage.

8. Fitting a gold crown or bridge.

9. Two surface amalgam restoration, after completion of the cavity preparation.

10. Taking primary alginate impressions for F/F dentures.

11. Taking an occlusal registration for F/F dentures.

12. To set up an anaesthetic machine ready, prior to use, for a dental general anaesthetic.

13. Testing the vitality of a tooth.

Short Essay Questions

Pathology, Microbiology and Sterilisation

1. What is inflammation, and what are its signs and symptoms?

2. Briefly relate the signs and symptoms of acute inflammation to what is happening in the tissues.

3. What are the major headings under which the causes of disease can be listed? Give examples under each heading.

4. How does the body resist infection?

5. Give the time cycle details of sterilising by water, steam and hot oven. What are the disadvantages of each method?

Anatomy and Physiology

6. Compare and contrast enamel and dentine.

7. In simple terms what is the mechanism of breathing?

8. In simple terms what is the mechanism of gaseous exchange in the capillaries?

9. What are the functions of the blood?

10. Describe the neuro-muscular events which follow treading, bare-footed on a pin.

11. What are the five main stages in the digestive process? Briefly indicate what happens at each stage.

Instruments, Materials and Drugs

12. How should surgical scissors be cared for? Give reasons.

13. What types of mouth props are there? Give examples and their uses.

14. How is slab impression compound made ready for use?

15. Briefly state the properties of the ideal dental filling material.

16. How should drugs used in dentistry be cared for?

17. There are four main routes of administration of drugs used in connection with dentistry. Name them, giving one example of each.

Dental Disease

18. What clinical, epidemiological and experimental evidence is available to associate refined carbohydrate with dental caries?

19. What advice can be given to children regarding sweet eating?

20. What are the consequences of a deepening periodontal pocket?

21. Name the types of calculus. What are the differences between them?

22. Patients sometimes say that a badly decayed tooth ached severely for a day or so and then suddenly the pain disappeared. What is the explanation?

23. How can caries be arrested?

24. There are two main processes in dental caries. Name each and state briefly what occurs in each.

25. Why is it important to clean the teeth properly after the last food and drink at night?

Restorative Dentistry

26. List the instruments and materials which should be laid out for a direct impression of an occlusal inlay cavity. Briefly give reasons for each item.

27. How may the D.A. assist the Dental Surgeon when a change of root dressing is being carried out?

28. How can a D.A. be helpful at the chairside during the dental treatment of children?

29. How can a D.A. avoid mercury contamination, and what precautions can she take when preparing amalgam for a filling?

30. How should a spillage of mercury be dealt with?

Anaesthesia, First Aid and Minor Oral Surgery

31. Local anaesthesia has several advantages over general anaesthesia. State some of these advantages.

32. What is the mechanism by which general anaesthetics take effect?

33. What are the duties of a D.A. during a general anaesthetic?

34. What are the duties of the D.A. during a patient's recovery from a general anaesthetic?

35. Describe how mouth-to-mouth resuscitation should be carried out. How can this technique be varied in the surgery?

36. Describe how external cardiac massage should be carried out on an adult. Briefly explain the technique.

37. How should fainting be treated? Give reasons for each part of the treatment.

38. Briefly list the duties of a D.A. before, during and after any minor oral surgery procedure.

Multiple Choice Questions

General

1. What is the name for a collection of similar cells grouped together with a special function?
   a) Organism
   b) Organ
   c) Gland
   d) Tissue
   e) System.

2. Which component of the blood is responsible for transporting oxygen?
   a) Red cells
   b) White cells
   c) Plasma
   d) Phagocytes
   e) Platelets.

3. Where does the digestion of starch begin?
   a) Mouth
   b) Oesophagus
   c) Stomach
   d) Duodenum
   e) Ileum.

4. The normal adult resting rate of respiration is
   a) 48
   b) 98
   c) 72
   d) 15
   e) 37.

5. The normal resting adult pulse rate is
   a) 37
   b) 16
   c) 70
   d) 98
   e) 104.

6. A scald is caused by
   a) Wet heat
   b) Dry heat
   c) Both
   d) Neither.

7. When does secondary haemorrhage occur?
   a) Immediately a tooth is extracted
   b) About 4 hours after extraction
   c) If the patient over-exercises
   d) When the local anaesthetic wears off
   e) If the socket becomes badly infected.

8. A prescription for barbiturate tablets should
   a) Be written and signed by a qualified D.A.
   b) Have the patient's name and address only written by a D.A.
   c) Be written by a D.A. and signed by a Dental Surgeon
   d) Only be written and signed by a Dental Surgeon.

9. An analgesic is a drug which
   a) Prevents infection
   b) Kills pain
   c) Prevents blood clotting
   d) Anaesthetises a patient.

10. The disadvantages of aspirin as an analgesic are
   a) The patient has to starve before taking aspirin
   b) It is too weak for dental pain
   c) It does not affect pulpitis
   d) It can cause gastric upsets.

11. Drugs of addiction should be stored
   a) In a refrigerator
   b) Out of the reach of children
   c) Upright in a drawer
   d) In a locked cupboard.

12. Whose responsibility is the care of drugs of addiction in a dental practice?
   a) The Dental Surgeon
   b) Any Dental Assistant
   c) The Senior Dental Assistant.

13. Fluoride is added to domestic water to produce a concentration very close to
   a) 100 parts per million
   b) 10 parts per million
   c) 4 parts per million
   d) 1 part per million.

14. Which important organ can be irreparably damaged by rheumatic fever?
   a) The tongue
   b) The liver
   c) The enamel organ
   d) The heart
   e) The spleen.

15. Subgingival calculus is always a feature of gingivitis
   a) True
   b) False.

16. The most frequently occurring disease of humans is
   a) Heart disease
   b) Cancer
   c) Dental caries
   d) Skin disease
   e) Arthritis.

17. Periodontitis is
   a) Inflammation of the pulp
   b) Dental caries
   c) Inflammation of the periodontal membrane
   d) Calculus
   e) Inflammation of the pericardium.

18. Occlusal registration means
   a) The occlusal surface of $\overline{8\,|\,8}$
   b) The bite stage in prosthetics
   c) An anterior occlusal radiograph
   d) The charting of occlusal cavities
   e) The construction of an obturator.

<u>Oral Anatomy</u>

19. A foramen is
   a) A prominent part of a bone
   b) A hole in a bone
   c) A natural opening in a bone for the passage of nerves and blood vessels
   d) A groove in the tooth enamel.

20. Immediately posterior to the hard palate is the
   a) Tongue
   b) Soft palate
   c) Pharynx
   d) Larynx
   e) Uvula.

21. The mental foramen is situated in
   a) The temporal bone
   b) The hard palate
   c) The mandible
   d) The sulcus
   e) The soft palate.

22. The cranial nerve supplying the teeth and jaws is
   a) III
   b) IV
   c) V
   d) VI
   e) VII.

23. A sensory nerve is one which carries stimuli
   a) From the peripheral tissues
   b) To the peripheral tissues
   c) To the muscles.

24. Ophthalmic, maxillary, mandibular are divisions of which cranial nerve?
   a) I
   b) II
   c) VII
   d) III
   e) V.

25. The nerve to the upper jaw is
   a) Sensory
   b) Motor
   c) Sensory and motor.

26. The mandibular nerve is
   a) Sensory
   b) Motor
   c) Sensory and motor.

27. The nerves usually affected when a mandibular nerve block is given are
   a) Anterior superior dental
   b) Long sphenopalatine
   c) Occlusal and buccal
   d) Intra osseous
   e) Inferior dental and lingual.

28. Name the folds of tissue which attach the gum in the mid-line to the lips
   a) Mandibular frenum
   b) Maxillary flange
   c) Lingual frenum
   d) Buccal frenum
   e) Labial frenae.

29. The tongue is mainly composed of
   a) Bone and muscle
   b) Gristle and muscle
   c) Adipose tissue
   d) Muscle fibres.

30. Select from List I the word most appropriate to each phrase in List II.

   List I

   a) Osteoblasts
   b) Fissures
   c) Contact points
   d) Incise
   e) Occlusal
   f) Palatal
   g) Odontoblasts
   h) Tear

   List II

   1) The prime function of incisor teeth is to ......
   2) The prime function of canine teeth is to ......
   3) The cells which form dentine are called ......
   4) Between the cusps of the posterior teeth lie the ......
   5) The cuspal surface of a molar tooth is called the ...... surface.

31. Select from List I the word most appropriate to each phrase in List II.

   List I

   a) Amelodentinal
   b) Gingivitis
   c) Apex
   d) Incisal edge
   e) Cusp
   f) Amelocemental
   g) Periodontitis
   h) Grind
   i) Periodontal
   j) Pericoronitis

List II

1) The prime function of posterior teeth is to ......
2) Inflammation around the crown of an erupting tooth is called ......
3) The tip of a tooth root is the ......
4) The visible junction of the crown and root is called the ...... junction
5) The biting part of an incisor tooth is the ......

32. Match the words in List I with the conditions in List II.

List I

a) Crown
b) Mesial
c) Resorption
d) Root
e) Distal
f) Occlusal
g) Absorption
h) Lingual
i) Impaction
j) Buccal.

List II

1) Obstruction to the eruption of a tooth
2) Shortening of the root of a deciduous tooth prior to natural loss
3) The parts of a tooth
4) The surfaces of a tooth.

33. An edentulous patient is one
a) With all his teeth
b) With no teeth
c) With no natural teeth
d) Who is unable to eat.

34. The components of dentine are
a) Calcium salts only
b) Calcium salts and some living cytoplasm
c) Calcium salts and blood vessels
d) Calcium salts and hollow tubules
e) Nerve endings and calcium salts.

35. The tooth is held in its socket by
a) Cementum
b) Bone
c) Periodontal membrane
d) The gum.

36. The maximum number of teeth usually found in the mouth of the human adult is
a) 20
b) 28
c) 24
d) 32
e) 36.

37. When a tooth erupts the root
a) Is fully formed
b) Is partly formed
c) Canal is closed
d) Canal is open
e) No cementum has formed.

38. Enamel is produced by
   a) Schwann cells
   b) Osteocytes
   c) Odontoblasts
   d) Lacunae
   e) Ameloblasts.

39. The roots of permanent teeth are completely formed
   a) When they erupt
   b) Six months after eruption
   c) About one year after eruption
   d) About two years after eruption
   e) About three years after eruption.

40. What is the maximum number of teeth usually found in the mouth of a four year old child?
   a) 16
   b) 20
   c) 24
   d) 32.

41. Which teeth do not have deciduous predecessors?
   a) Molars
   b) Premolars
   c) Canines
   d) Incisors.

42. What is the usual sequence of eruption of deciduous teeth?
   a) a b c d e
   b) a c b d e
   c) a b d c e
   d) a b c e d
   e) a c b e d.

43. Incisor teeth are those which are
   a) Chisel-shaped cutting teeth
   b) Sharp tearing teeth
   c) Large grinding teeth
   d) Ridged crushing teeth
   e) Pointed flesh shearing teeth.

44. Taste buds are found mainly on
   a) Tongue
   b) Cheek
   c) Soft palate
   d) Hard palate
   e) Lips.

45. A diastema is
   a) An unerupted tooth
   b) A supernumerary tooth
   c) A type of orthodontic appliance
   d) The surgical removal of a buried root
   e) A wide space between two adjacent teeth.

46. What is the name given to the fold of tissue attached to the floor of the mouth between the openings of the sub-mandibular glands?
   a) Labial frenum
   b) Buccal frenum
   c) Mandibular frenum
   d) Palatal frenum
   e) Lingual frenum.

47. A normal healthy tongue should be
a) Smooth and shiny
b) Furred and grey
c) White and smooth
d) Red and shiny
e) Pink and roughened.

Microbiology

48. Examples of bacteria are
a) Yeasts
b) Viruses
c) Bacilli
d) Cocci.

49. For growth, micro-organisms do not need
a) Sunlight
b) Moisture
c) Carbohydrate and protein
d) Suitable temperature.

50. In very adverse conditions what happens to most viruses?
a) They die
b) They cease to multiply
c) They form spores
d) They become quiescent.

51. What are the main ways of killing micro-organisms on dental instruments?
a) Flaming
b) Immersion in antiseptics
c) Irradiation
d) Sterilisation.

52. All spores can be killed by
a) Chlorhexidine 20% solution in water
b) Autoclave for 3 minutes at 134°C
c) Boiling water for one hour
d) Neat Dettol
e) Dry heat for one hour at 160°C.

53. A true sterilisation cycle is:-
a) Steam at 126°C for 18 minutes
b) Hot air at 120°C for two hours
c) Water at 100°C for 10 minutes.

54. After removal from the steriliser, dental forceps should be
a) Placed in water to cool
b) Stored in disinfectant
c) Dried on a towel
d) Stored in a sterile container
e) Stored in a surgery drawer.

55. The best method of cleaning hands in the surgery is
a) Wash in chlorhexidine for 2 minutes
b) Scrub with antiseptic soap for 5 minutes
c) Wash with antiseptic soap then with industrial spirit
d) Wash with hot water and dry in hot air
e) Scrub with hot water and dry on a hand towel.

56. Which organism is most likely to lead to which condition?

1) Streptococci	a) Denture sore mouth
2) Salmonella	b) Sore throat
3) Treponema	c) Boils
4) Pneumococci	d) Acute ulcerative gingivitis
5) Lactobacillus	
6) Fungi	
7) Staphylococci	
8) Bacillus coli.	

Materials

57. For accuracy, both the alginate powder and the water for mixing should be at a temperature of
   a) 37°C
   b) 37°F
   c) 70°F
   d) 98°F.

58. Hydrocolloid impression materials are
   a) Irreversible
   b) Reversible
   c) Both
   d) Neither.

59. If an alginate impression cannot be cast immediately it should be
   a) Stored in water
   b) Left to dry, then placed in a bag
   c) Wrapped in a damp cloth and placed in a polythene bag
   d) Coated with thin oil
   e) Placed in a refrigerator.

60. After removal from the mouth, an alginate impression should be washed to
   a) Remove saliva and food debris
   b) Sharpen detail on the impression
   c) Cool the impression
   d) Stop chemical reactions in the alginate
   e) Complete the setting.

61. Which is correct? Plaster of Paris
   a) Originally came from the ground under Paris
   b) Models can be ground for re-use
   c) Is never used in the mouth
   d) Has to be mixed with a special plastic to make it harden.

62. Pink wax sheets are normally used in dentistry for
   a) Wax forms of gold inlay cavities
   b) Protecting models
   c) Locating denture over-extension
   d) Protecting new silicate fillings
   e) Occlusal registration.

63. Plaster of Paris is used to take impressions for
a) Bridges
b) Partial dentures
c) Reline of full dentures
d) Orthodontic appliances
e) New full dentures.

64. Soft linings are used in dentistry
a) Under porcelain crowns
b) In deep cavities
c) On the fitting surfaces of dentures
d) Under silicate fillings
e) In trays to store sharp instruments.

65. Materials which are added to the periphery of special trays to produce a functional edge fit are
a) Composition
b) Peripheral seal
c) Gutta percha
d) Alginate
e) Sticky wax.

66. Which materials are rarely used on their own for full denture reline impressions?
a) Rubber base
b) Zinc oxide/Eugenol paste
c) Resilient lining material
d) Viscogel
e) Peripheral seal.

67. The base of a full denture is usually made from
a) Stainless steel
b) Acrylic
c) Vulcanite
d) Gold
e) Silver.

68. Which materials are not used to make denture teeth?
a) Plastic
b) Porcelain
c) Gold
d) Stainless steel
e) Vulcanite.

69. A tissue conditioner is
a) A powder sprinkled on to a denture's fitting surface
b) A powder/liquid cream applied to a denture's fitting surface
c) A wax which is soft at mouth temperature
d) A constituent of alginate powder.

70. Gutta percha is
a) A rubber material
b) A man-made plastic
c) Used for mouth impressions
d) Used as a soft lining
e) Used as a temporary denture.

Prosthetics

71. Prosthesis means
   a) Oral hygiene instruction
   b) The application of topical fluoride
   c) A general anaesthetic
   d) An artificial replacement for lost tissue
   e) Calcification of teeth.

72. Loose, ill-fitting full dentures can cause
   a) Ulceration of the mouth
   b) Excessive wear of the fitting surface
   c) Problems in making new dentures
   d) The dentures to become coated with calculus
   e) The tongue to grow bigger.

73. Which of the following materials is suitable on its own for final full denture impressions?
   a) Alginate
   b) Composition sheets
   c) Composition sticks
   d) Plaster of Paris
   e) Gutta percha.

74. When a plaster of Paris impression is removed from the mouth it may break. The pieces should be
   a) Thrown away
   b) Put aside for the Dental Surgeon to deal with
   c) Put in a bag and sent to the laboratory.

75. An alginate impression mix should be well spatulated in order to
   a) Mix the powder with the water
   b) Reduce air bubbles
   c) Slow down the setting time
   d) Include air
   e) Speed up setting time.

76. The reason for the holes in impression trays is to
   a) Allow escape of excess impression material
   b) Reduce the weight of the tray
   c) Allow the escape of air trapped in the impression material
   d) Allow the dentist to see when the tray is finally seated
   e) Anchor the impression material.

77. Materials commonly used for final impressions for partial dentures are
   a) Plaster of Paris
   b) Composition
   c) Alginate
   d) Rubber base
   e) Zinc Oxide/Eugenol.

78. A patient brings in a lower partial denture with a broken lingual bar. This can be accepted for repair without reference to a Dental Surgeon.
a) True   b) False.

79. The objective at the impression stage for full dentures is to
a) Reproduce the shape of the patient's jaws
b) Obtain a print of the denture-bearing area and adjacent tissues
c) Obtain a model of the hard and soft tissues of the mouth
d) Obtain a model of the jaws.

80. The main objective in taking an impression in a special tray is to
a) Obtain a better peripheral outline
b) Cover the maximum gingival surface
c) Obtain an accurate impression of all the denture-bearing tissues
d) Reduce the number of eases of the full denture.

81. During construction of full dentures, the objective at the bite stage is to record
a) The relationship of the patient's dental arches to the skull
b) The vertical space between the patient's jaws
c) The vertical and anteroposterior relationship of the patient's jaws
d) The position of the teeth
e) In wax the patient's "bite".

82. In the construction of full dentures, some of the objectives at the try-in stage are to check
a) The number of teeth
b) The fit of the denture
c) The peripheral outline
d) The shade of the wax
e) The vertical dimension.

83. The objective at the fit stage of full dentures is
a) Only to give the patient his dentures
b) To check the fit and to carry out any necessary occlusal grinding
c) To ease sore spots
d) Only to fit the dentures and to check appearance.

84. Patient instructions in the care of acrylic full dentures should include
a) Regular cleaning in a mild detergent
b) Always to wear them at night
c) Regular cleaning with an abrasive
d) Not to drink hot drinks
e) Cleaning over a bowl of water.

85. When full dentures are worn the jaws
   a) No longer shrink
   b) Shrink more rapidly
   c) Change more at the back of the mouth
   d) Change more at the front of the mouth
   e) Shrink fairly evenly and slowly.

86. For most older patients full dentures should be replaced at least every
   a) One year
   b) Three years
   c) Ten years
   d) Twenty five years.

87. The appearance of an edentulous patient can be improved if the full dentures have
   a) The correct position of the anterior teeth
   b) Correct thickness of the acrylic flanges
   c) Correct vertical dimensions
   d) Light coloured teeth
   e) Small upper incisor teeth.

88. A patient brings in a full acrylic denture with the upper right labial flange missing. This can be repaired without an impression
   a) True
   b) False.

89. A broken vulcanite denture should not be accepted for repair without reference to the Dental Surgeon because
   a) It cannot be repaired
   b) An impression is always required
   c) Only some types can be repaired
   d) It is better repaired in the mouth
   e) A new denture may be necessary.

90. The selection of artificial teeth for a replacement for full dentures depends upon
   a) The patient's complexion
   b) The size, shape and colour of the patient's natural teeth
   c) The size of the patient's face
   d) The time the patient has been without natural teeth
   e) The space between the patient's dental arches.

Radiography

91. A safelight may be tested in the dark room by
   a) An exposure meter
   b) Placing an open film beneath the lamp
   c) Placing a coin on an open film beneath the lamp
   d) Placing an open film in the dark room for two minutes
   e) None of these.

UNIVERSITY COLLEGE CORK Library

92. Undue exposure of X-ray film to dark room safelight leads to
a) No change
b) Blurred image
c) Fogging
d) Mottling.

93. Which films are not used intra-orally?
a) Periapical
b) Interproximal
c) Occlusal
d) Pan-oral
e) Bi-molar.

94. To reduce radiation hazards to the patient
a) The patient should wear a lead apron
b) Children should not be radiographed
c) Slow films should be used
d) Routine films should not be repeated within one year
e) Rapid developer should be used.

95. To reduce radiation hazards to herself the D.A. should
a) Never hold the film in the patient's mouth
b) Stand beside the patient
c) Avoid retakes
d) Hold the film in the patient's mouth using artery forceps
e) Get the patient to operate the timing switch.

96. A shorter exposure time is required for lower incisors than for upper molars because
a) The teeth are smaller
b) The X-ray tube is further away
c) The film is closer to the X-ray tube
d) The angle of the tube to tooth is greater.

97. The light and dark parts on a radiograph are due to
a) Different absorption levels by the object
b) Extra radiation given off by the object
c) Varied exposure time
d) The method of developing
e) Variations in emulsion thickness.

98. A bite wing radiograph will indicate to the Dental Surgeon
a) Interstitial caries
b) Calculus
c) Interdental bone crest
d) The periapical condition
e) Incisal caries.

99. A periapical radiograph is primarily taken to indicate to a Dental Surgeon
a) Root morphology
b) Non-vital teeth
c) Interstitial caries
d) Salivary calculus
e) Enamel thickness.

100. Bimolar or oblique lateral radiographs are primarily taken to show
- a) Fractures and swellings of the jaws
- b) The development of unerupted teeth
- c) Bone loss in periodontal disease
- d) Interstitial caries
- e) A root in the antrum.

101. An occlusal radiograph is primarily taken to show
- a) The presence and position of unerupted teeth
- b) Submandibular salivary gland calculus
- c) A root in the antrum
- d) Caries in anterior teeth
- e) The length of incisor roots.

102. A cassette and an intensifying screen are necessary for which films?
- a) Orthopantomogram
- b) Bimolar
- c) Bite wing
- d) Lower occlusal
- e) Periapical.

103. Orthopantomograms are not usually taken to show
- a) Presence and position of unerupted teeth
- b) Early interstitial caries
- c) Bone loss in periodontal disease
- d) Periapical abnormalities.

104. Excess radiation may be reduced by
- a) Using fast films
- b) Using extra-oral films
- c) Increasing the distance between the X-ray cone and the patient
- d) Using a small aperture.

105. Which tissues are most likely to be damaged by radiation?
- a) Hair and skin
- b) Blood cells
- c) Reproductive organs
- d) Nerves
- e) Bone.

106. Which of the following is not an intra-oral film?
- a) Bite wing
- b) Periapical
- c) Bimolar
- d) Orthopantomograph
- e) Occlusal.

107. What is the usual range of temperature for developer?
- a) 168-175°F
- b) 37-40°C
- c) 68-70°C
- d) 68-75°F.

108. The reason for washing an X-ray film between developing stages is to
- a) Aid chemical reaction
- b) Remove unwanted chemicals
- c) Remove fingerprints
- d) To prevent over-development of the films.

109. The reasons for "fixing" a film are to

a) Prevent streaking
b) Sharpen the image
c) Produce a matt finish
d) Remove chemicals in the film.

110. Match the faulty radiograph state in List I with the likely causes in List II.

List I

a) Yellowing of radiograph
b) Herringbone pattern on radiograph
c) Mottling.

List II

1) Developer too warm
2) Air bubbles in tanks
3) Film in mouth the wrong way around
4) Film damaged by bending
5) Big temperature difference between tanks
6) Insufficient rinsing after fixing.

111. Match the faulty radiograph state in List I with the likely causes in List II.

List I

a) Very dark picture
b) Blurred image
c) Partial image.

List II

1) Too long in the developer
2) Developer not warm enough
3) X-ray tube not properly lined up
4) Film moved
5) Over-exposure to radiation
6) Insufficient rinsing
7) Film in contact with another in developing tank
8) Patient moved
9) Developer too warm
10) Faulty safelight.

Anaesthesia

112. Name two basic techniques of administering local anaesthetic

a) Infiltration
b) Intravenous
c) Intramuscular
d) Perineural
e) Inhalation.

113. Select from List I the most appropriate word to complete sentences in List II.

List I

a) Sensory
b) Motor
c) Central
d) Peripheral
e) Anaesthesia
f) Analgesia.

List II

1) Painful sensations pass along ...... nerves to the brain
2) To move away from pain, the muscles receive impulses from the brain along ...... nerves
3) Interruption of painful impulses to the brain by means of chemicals is called ......

114. Dental Surgeons are mainly concerned with pain sensations in which cranial nerves?
a) III
b) V
c) VI
d) VIII
e) X.

115. Local anaesthetic can aid in the diagnosis of the causes of pain
a) True
b) False.

116. An ideal local anaesthetic compound should have which of the following properties?
a) It works quickly
b) It wears off quickly
c) It spread quickly
d) It irritates tissues
e) It can be sterilised.

117. A slight colouring of the local anaesthetic solution
a) Is normal
b) Should be reported to the Dental Surgeon
c) Indicates that the solution should be thrown away
d) Occurs in stronger solutions
e) Occurs if the solution is too warm.

118. Precautions may be necessary when local anaesthetic solutions containing adrenalin are used if the patient is taking
a) Analgesics
b) Some antibiotics
c) Antihistamines
d) Certain anti-depressant drugs
e) Cortico-steroid drugs.

119. Failure to obtain local anaesthesia may be due to
a) Out of date solution
b) Too much vaso-constrictor
c) Weak anaesthetic
d) Faulty technique
e) A blunt needle.

120. Administering an infiltration local anaesthetic causes the tissues to swell
a) False   b) True.

121. The main reason why a disposable cartridge needle should not be re-sterilised is because
a) It may be blunt
b) It may break
c) The plastic would melt
d) The plastic sleeve cannot be resealed
e) Sterility cannot be guaranteed.

122. The strength of adrenalin in local anaesthetic solutions is
a) 1 in 100
b) 1 in 1000
c) 1 in 80
d) 1 in 80,000
e) 1 in 10,000.

123. Give two reasons why vaso-constrictors are present in local anaesthetic solutions
a) To sterilise the solution
b) To prolong the anaesthetic time
c) Reduce haemorrhage
d) Make the anaesthetic work faster
e) Strengthen the anaesthetic.

124. Sedative drugs are a substitute for a local anaesthetic
a) True   b) False.

125. Indicate which types of local anaesthetic technique is most likely to be used in each case
a) Regional
b) Infiltration
c) Topical

1) Extraction of both lower canines
2) Cavity preparation in lower molars
3) Pulpotomy of upper pre-molars
4) Taking a copper ring impression
5) Gingivectomy round lower incisors
6) Apicectomy in upper lateral incisor.

126. Partially used local anaesthetic cartridges can be used again
a) True   b) False.

127. Match the words in List I with the descriptions in List II

List I

a) Intraneural
b) Infiltration
c) Topical
d) General
e) Trigeminal
f) Regional nerve block.

List II

1) An anaesthetic drug applied to the surface of the skin or to mucosa
2) An anaesthetic drug applied adjacent to a nerve trunk
3) An anaesthetic drug applied adjacent to the site of operation
4) An anaesthetic drug applied at some point along a nerve
5) An anaesthetic drug injected into a vein and carried to the brain.

128. Anaesthesia means loss of
a) All sensation
b) Consciousness
c) Pain sensation.

129. Analgesia means
a) Loss of all sensation
b) State of unconsciousness
c) Loss of pain sensation
d) A type of drug.

130. Nitrous oxide is supplied in a cylinder coloured
a) Red
b) Black with white collar
c) Orange
d) Blue
e) Grey.

131. What is meant by cyanosis?
a) Blueness of skin usually associated with oxygen lack
b) A poisonous chemical in the blood
c) Discolouration of nitrous oxide gas
d) Excess CO_2 in the blood
e) Condition due to excessive alcohol intake.

132. Which drug can be added to nitrous oxide/oxygen mixture to produce a smoother anaesthetic?
a) Halothane
b) Methohexitone
c) Haloperidol
d) Trytyline
e) Methane.

133. The minimum percentage of oxygen normally given with nitrous oxide as an anaesthetic is
a) 5%
b) 10%
c) 0%
d) 20%
e) 25%.

134. Premedication is
   a) Thinking about a future event
   b) Given to relieve after-pain
   c) To help a patient recover from a general anaesthetic
   d) Sterilisation of the mucosa before giving an injection
   e) Used to allay a patient's fears.

135. The main disadvantage of oral premedication is
   a) A very high dosage is needed
   b) There is variable absorption from the stomach
   c) The bitter taste
   d) The patient has to be starved
   e) Patient's dislike injections.

136. Three hours after the injection of a sedation dose of Diazepam most patients
   a) Would be asleep
   b) Would be fit to drive a car
   c) Could return home with an escort
   d) Could return to work.

<u>Caries</u>

137. Early enamel decay shows clinically as
   a) An opaque white patch
   b) Chipping of the enamel
   c) A brown patch
   d) A radiopaque area.

138. Enamel caries differs from dentine caries because dentine
   a) Has a higher temperature
   b) Is not bathed in saliva
   c) Has a blood supply
   d) Has no nerve supply
   e) Has a greater organic content.

139. Caries occurs mainly in fissures and interdental spaces because they are
   a) Areas of weak dentine
   b) Difficult areas for the Dental Surgeon to examine
   c) Never in contact with saliva
   d) Difficult areas to clean properly
   e) Areas of weak enamel.

140. Dental caries occurs in soft tissues
   a) True
   b) False.

141. Dental caries always starts
   a) Externally
   b) Internally
   c) Both.

142. Dental caries does not occur in
   a) Unerupted teeth
   b) Partially erupted teeth
   c) Fully erupted teeth only
   d) The pulp
   e) Supernumerary teeth.

143. The carious process
- a) Is bacteria converting carbohydrates to acids
- b) Is acid foods attacking the enamel
- c) Is bacteria eroding the enamel
- d) Is plaque attacking the enamel
- e) Involves proteolysis and decalcification.

144. When caries has passed through enamel it spreads primarily
- a) Along the amelodentinal junction
- b) Into the pulp
- c) Into dentine
- d) Into cementum.

145. Food is more likely to stagnate around teeth which are
- a) Unopposed
- b) Unerupted
- c) Irregular
- d) Crowned
- e) Spaced.

146. Research work has shown that the greatest incidence of dental caries is associated with
- a) Sticky sugar as a part of each meal
- b) Sugary drinks at mealtimes
- c) Sugar intake between meals.

147. The commonest cause of a dental abscess in young people is
- a) Gum disease
- b) Injury
- c) Erupting teeth
- d) Pulp death.

148. Toothache is associated with
- a) Enamel decay
- b) Exposed interdental bone
- c) Pulp exposure
- d) Exposed cementum
- e) Early dentine decay.

149. The pulp tries to protect itself against a low grade caries process by
- a) Increasing its blood supply
- b) Forming secondary dentine
- c) Forming an abscess
- d) Recording painful sensations
- e) None of these.

150. Pulpal necrosis means
- a) Chronic inflammation of the pulp
- b) A healthy pulp
- c) Partial removal of the pulp
- d) Total removal of the pulp
- e) Death of the pulp.

151. Dental caries means loss of tooth substance due to
- a) Bacteria
- b) Chemicals in the mouth
- c) Sweets
- d) Food and bacteria
- e) The enamel crumbling.

Children's Dentistry

152. Orthodontics is mainly concerned with
a) Maladjustment
b) Malocclusion
c) Mastication
d) Articulation.

153. A removable orthodontic appliance usually needs to be adjusted by the Dental Surgeon once
a) A day
b) A week
c) A month
d) Every three months.

154. A supernumerary tooth means
a) An incisor tooth
b) An extra tooth
c) An unusually shaped tooth
d) A type of posterior tooth.

155. Early loss of deciduous teeth can allow the space for the premolars to close
a) True
b) False.

156. The primary aim of orthodontics is to enable a patient to
a) Have a reduced caries rate
b) Keep his teeth clean
c) Talk properly
d) Bite with the teeth in any position
e) Have well-aligned teeth.

157. Crowding usually means that the patient has
a) Too many teeth
b) Canines which are erupting buccally
c) Insufficient space for the third premolars
d) The correct number of teeth
e) Larger teeth than the jaws can accommodate.

158. Prolonged retention of deciduous teeth can lead to two rows of teeth
a) True
b) False.

159. Large jaws together with small teeth lead to overcrowding
a) True
b) False.

160. A patient with a damaged removable orthodontic appliance should
a) See his Dental Surgeon as soon as possible
b) See his Dental Surgeon within a week
c) Wait until his next appointment
d) Continue to wear it if possible
e) Leave it out immediately.

161. A loose band on a fixed orthodontic appliance should be pushed back into place and left until the next appointment
a) True
b) False.

162. Stainless steel bands of a fixed orthodontic appliance are held in place by
a) Being a very tight fit
b) Cement
c) Neither of these
d) Both of these.

163. Removable orthodontic appliances should be taken out to be cleaned
a) Daily
b) After each meal
c) Before bed
d) Only by the Dental Surgeon.

164. Retained deciduous teeth and supernumerary teeth are possible causes of overcrowding
a) False
b) True.

165. Deciduous teeth can cause malformation of the permanent teeth
a) By infection
b) By pressure
c) By retention
d) By premature loss.

166. Deciduous teeth are not sensitive to pain
a) True
b) False.

167. The proportion of the pulp to the crown of a deciduous tooth compared to its permanent successor is
a) Greater
b) About the same
c) Smaller.

168. Deciduous teeth are not sensitive to pain from drilling
a) True
b) False.

169. A child has a temper tantrum in the surgery, the D.A. should
a) Slap the child's face
b) Play a quiet supportive role to the Dental Surgeon
c) Take over from the Dental Surgeon
d) Fetch the child's parent
e) None of these.

170. Deciduous teeth are seldom filled with
a) Amalgam
b) Composite
c) Gold
d) Copper amalgam
e) Porcelain.

171. Exposure of the pulp of an incisor tooth in a 7 year old child would be treated by
a) Pulpotomy
b) Pulpectomy
c) Neither
d) Both.

172. Endodontics can be carried out on deciduous teeth
a) True
b) False.

173. A blow to a permanent incisor tooth may result in the fracture of
a) The enamel
b) The dentine
c) The root
d) The alveolar bone
e) The pulp.

174. A permanent incisor which has been knocked out cleanly
a) Can never be replaced in its socket
b) Can sometimes be replaced in its socket
c) Has to be cemented into the socket
d) Has to be crowned before replacing it in its socket.

175. A Dental Surgeon would be more likely to carry out a pulpotomy on an incisor of a 7 year old because
a) The dentine is very sensitive
b) There is not yet a nerve in the root of the tooth
c) The cement has not formed
d) The pulp chamber is too small
e) The root apex is open.

176. A young patient who has received a blow to a permanent central incisor should be
a) Given an appointment within 24 hours if possible
b) Told not to bother until his next regular check up
c) Asked to make an appointment if the pain persists after one week
d) Advised to attend the local hospital
e) Advised to see his medical practitioner.

<u>Conservation</u>

177. Briault, sickle, pocket measuring, are examples of
a) Paper points
b) Locking tweezers
c) Scalers
d) Probes
e) Spatulae.

178. A "high" dental restoration will
a) Increase biting efficiency
b) Increase chances of fracture of the restoration
c) Make the opposing teeth tender
d) Allow for wear of the restoration
e) Not matter.

179. "White" fillings are seldom used to fill cavities in posterior teeth because part of the material
a) Reacts adversely with premolar and molar enamel
b) Is difficult to use
c) Wears away easily
d) Takes too long to set
e) Creeps under occlusal stress.

180. Amalgam is retained in a cavity due to
   a) The cavity's shape
   b) The cavity lining
   c) Adherence to cavity wall
   d) Enamel cement.

181. Amalgam when inserted into a cavity is said to be "plastic". This means that it is
   a) Soft and able to be handled
   b) Made from acrylic or similar resins
   c) Both
   d) Neither.

182. Immediately after insertion amalgam should be
   a) Carved
   b) Burnished
   c) Polished
   d) Triturated
   e) Varnished.

183. Amalgam is usually preferred to gold as a posterior filling material because of its
   a) Strength
   b) Appearance
   c) Better cavity retention
   d) Ease of use.

184. The reasons for condensing amalgam fillings are
   a) To exclude moisture
   b) To reduce the amount of mercury in the amalgam
   c) To strengthen the amalgam
   d) To minimise porosity
   e) To adhere the amalgam to the enamel.

185. If the automatic amalgam mixer breaks down, you could mix amalgam using
   a) A rubber finger stall
   b) The palm of the hand and a finger
   c) An empty tablet bottle in which to shake it
   d) A mortar and pestle
   e) There is no alternative method.

186. Amalgam fillings are carved in order to
   a) Reduce the weight of the filling
   b) To aid mastication
   c) To reduce breakage
   d) To strengthen the filling
   e) Speed the setting of amalgam.

187. Polishing of fillings
   a) Reduces the chance of further decay
   b) Makes the filling look better
   c) Removes mercury
   d) Strengthens the filling
   e) Removes marginal ledges.

188. Mixed amalgam should not be mulled in the hand because
- a) It makes the hands dirty
- b) It may absorb moisture from the hands
- c) Mercury may be absorbed by the skin
- d) It speeds the setting time
- e) It slows the setting time.

189. A Dental Surgeon takes a radiograph of a traumatised permanent central incisor to
- a) Check for a root fracture
- b) See if the apex of the root is open or closed
- c) See if the pulp is broken
- d) Check the vitality of the tooth
- e) Determine the length of the root canal.

190. Match the names in List I with the descriptions in List II

List I

- a) Mummification
- b) Pulpotomy
- c) Coronectomy
- d) Pulpectomy
- e) Devitalisation
- f) Necrosis
- g) Polypus.

List II

- 1) Complete removal of pulp
- 2) Partial removal of pulp
- 3) Death of the pulp
- 4) Preservation of a dead pulp.

191. Detailed impressions of a jacket crown preparation are obtained using
- a) Irreversible hydrocolloids
- b) Rubber impression materials
- c) Zinc oxide paste
- d) Brown stick composition
- e) Reversible hydrocolloids.

192. Examples of an impression material elastic at room temperature are
- a) Silicone or rubber base material
- b) Composition
- c) Alginate
- d) Reversible hydrocolloid
- e) Zinc oxide/Eugenol.

193. Gold shell crowns are fabricated in the laboratory by
- a) Machine pressing
- b) Bending by hand
- c) Casting molten metal into high temperature moulds
- d) Carving from a block.

194. Porcelain jacket crowns are fabricated in a laboratory by
   a) Heating ceramic glass powder and water
   b) Casting porcelain at room temperature
   c) Pouring a soft porcelain dough into a mould
   d) Carving from a block of porcelain.

195. A jacket crown can best be defined as an
   a) Artificial replacement of tooth substance
   b) Artificial replacement of most of the visible tooth substance
   c) Artificial replacement of the enamel and dentine
   d) Artificial replacement of the enamel.

196. The crown preparations on the teeth supporting a bridge should
   a) Be parallel to each other
   b) Be parallel mesio-distally
   c) Converge
   d) Diverge.

197. Which material is not used in the construction of permanent crowns?
   a) Porcelain
   b) Gold
   c) Silver
   d) Acrylic
   e) Aluminium.

198. The shade of the labial face of a porcelain jacket crown is
   a) Even all over
   b) Darker at the neck
   c) Lighter at the mesial side
   d) Darker in the centre.

199. Which materials are commonly used to construct temporary anterior crowns?
   a) Epimines
   b) Composition
   c) Zinc oxide
   d) Zinc oxyphosphate
   e) Composites.

200. Which of the following words is not a type of crown?
   a) Post
   b) Shell
   c) Jacket
   d) Basket
   e) Bevel
   f) Three quarter.

201. Porcelain jacket crowns are seldom fitted for patients under 14 years of age because
   a) There is a risk of fracture
   b) The root will grow longer
   c) The clinical crown will alter
   d) The shade of adjacent teeth will alter.

202. Materials used to construct temporary posterior crowns are
   a) Stainless steel crown form
   b) Copper ring
   c) Celluloid crown form
   d) Zinc oxide/Eugenol
   e) Zinc phosphate cement
   f) Mouth curing acrylics
   g) Amalgam
   h) Gutta percha
   i) Aluminium crown form.

203. Which of the items listed should be laid out ready for use in taking copper ring impressions?
a) Red slab composition
b) Brown stick composition
c) Blue inlay wax
d) Tweezers
e) Crown scissors
f) Vaseline
g) Wire cutters
h) Selection of copper rings.

204. Crowns cannot be made on root filled teeth
a) True
b) False.

205. Detailed impressions for a bridge are usually obtained using
a) Alginate
b) Rubber impression material
c) Zinc oxide paste
d) Brown stick composition
e) Reversible hydrocolloid.

206. Which term is not normally applied to dental bridges
a) Suspension
b) Cantilever
c) Fixed-fixed
d) Fixed-free.

207. Select the materials used for permanent bridges
a) Gold
b) Acrylic
c) Chrome cobalt
d) Porcelain
e) Stainless steel.

208. Which of the following are important parts of a bridge?
a) Arch bar
b) Abutment
c) Crib
d) Pontic
e) Occlusal rest
f) Clasp
g) Lingual bar.

209. The majority of bridges are fixed to supporting teeth by means of crowns. This is because
a) There is no other means of supporting a bridge
b) This way the bridge is easier to construct in the laboratory
c) The bridge is less inclined to rotate
d) There is greater resistance to secondary caries.

210. The cement mix for fixing a bridge should
a) Drop from the spatula
b) Just fail to drop from the spatula
c) Be of a thick cream consistency
d) Be stiff.

PART 2
ANSWERS

UNIVERSITY COLLEGE
Library
CORK

Oro-Facial Anatomy

1. Left and right maxilla.

2. The maxillary antrum.

3. The palate.

4. Cleft palate.

5. The rounded posterior end of the maxillary alveolar bone.

6. A natural opening on the surface of a bone.

7. The spongy tooth bearing bone of both jaws.

8. The compact bone which remains after the extraction of teeth and the healing of the sockets.

9. Coronoid process - attachment of the temporalis muscle. Condyle - articulation with the base of the skull. It forms part of the temporo-mandibular joint.

10. The inferior dental foramen. It allows the passage of the inferior dental nerve and blood vessels.

11. Between the apices of the lower premolar teeth.

12. The mouth is open and will not close. The mandible is protruded.

13. It has a layer of keratinised (toughened) cells, which masks the vascular redness.

14. a) Rugae.
    b) It is a mucoperiosteum.

15. To close the nasal cavity from the mouth, so preventing food and liquids getting into the nose. It aids speech.

16. Between the alveolus and the cheek.

17. The mucous membrane.

18. In mastication and swallowing. As an organ of sensation. In speech.

19. Parotid - in front of the ear. Submandibular - inside the angle of the mandible. Sublingual - under the anterior part of the floor of the mouth.

20. Protection, lubrication, cleansing, aid to speech, digestion of starch.

21. Decrease can be due to disease, nervousness, or some drugs. Increase can be due to the sight or smell of food, teething, or objects in the mouth.

22. Mumps.

23. Temporalis masseter and medial pterygoid muscles.

24. The lateral pterygoid.

25. Muscles of facial expression.

26. It forms the floor of the mouth and can cause a lower denture to lift off the alveolar ridge.

27. The mandibular division of trigeminal nerve, cranial V.

28. V or trigeminal. Ophthalmic, maxillary, mandibular.

29. The mental branch of the mandibular nerve - a branch of cranial V, the trigeminal nerve.

30. The lingual nerve, a branch of the mandibular nerve runs close by the inferior dental foramen. The anaesthetic solution will in consequence usually affect the lingual nerve.

31. a) Inferior dental block, to anaesthetise the tooth and lingual gum.
    b) Buccal infiltration to anaesthetise the long buccal nerve which innervates the buccal gum.

32. This bone is very dense and an infiltration anaesthetic would produce very little anaesthesia of the teeth; therefore a regional anaesthetic is given.

33. Anterior palatine, naso-palatine, posterior, middle and anterior superior dental.

34. a) The infra mandibular muscles relax.
    b) The muscles of mastication contract.

35. Periosteum.

Tooth Anatomy

1. a) Labial — d) Buccal
   b) Lingual — e) Mesial
   c) Palatal — f) Distal

2. A group of tissues from which a tooth develops.

3. Six months after birth.

4. Deciduous teeth a) have more bulbous crowns
   b) are smaller and whiter
   c) have divergent molar roots.

5. a) Incisors
   b) Canines
   c) Second molars
   d) First molars
   e) Upper first molars
   f) Upper canines and central incisors
   g) Lower incisors
   h) Lower molars and upper first premolars
   i) Upper molars
   j) Occasionally lower 6's.

6. To allow space for the permanent successors to develop.

7. A and D.

8. Premolars.

9. Enamel, dentine and pulp.

10. Dentine, cementum and pulp.

11. By the periodontal membrane which is attached to the bone forming the socket.

12. Between the roots of a tooth.

13. At or near the apex of each root of each tooth.

14. A dentine forming cell.

15. On occlusal surfaces and at cusps.

16. The amelo-dentinal junction.

17. Rods or prisms of calcium salts.

18. Via dentinal tubules.

19. The periodontal membrane: to hold the tooth in position.

20. No. Dentine is sensitive.

21. Secondary dentine can be laid down, reducing the size of the pulp.

22. Nerves, blood vessels and connective tissue.

23. The area where two adjacent teeth touch. Usually only enamel is involved.

24. $\overline{1|1}$ or $\overline{6|6}$. Six years.

Pathology and Microbiology

1. a) One thousandth of a millimetre
   b) One millionth of a millimetre.

2. a) Direct contact, either person to person or person to instrument
   b) Droplet or particle, e.g. coughing or dust
   c) Animals including insects
   d) Liquids, e.g. milk.

3. Nutriments, moisture, lack of sunlight, correct temperature and correct level of oxygen.

4. Skin folds, under nails, on hair, in body openings and tracts.

5. Through body surfaces, e.g. respiratory or alimentary tracts, damaged skin, mucous membrane.

6. A carrier.

7. a) Whether the organism causes disease in a particular species
   b) The virulence of the organism
   c) The resistance of the individual.

8. Bacteraemia.

9. The individual's resistance to disease.

10. The Tetanus organisms release toxins from the local site of injury which lead to muscular contractions of distant muscles, e.g. of the masseter muscle.

11. Fungi (Candida Albicans).

12. a) Powerful chemical agents which destroy many living organisms as well as living tissue
    b) Chemical agents which inhibit the growth of microbes
    c) Drugs derived from living organisms which kill or inhibit the growth of other organisms.

13. To remove debris and micro organisms; this will reduce cross infections.

14. Septicaemia.

15. It is a thick creamy-yellow liquid containing:
    a) white cells - dead and dying
    b) organisms - dead and living
    c) necrotic tissue cells.

16. An abscess.

17. Healthy patients are resistant to most of their own micro organisms.

18. Serum hepatitis.

19. The patient's defence response may be high and/or the cause may be very mild.

20. a) Remove the cause: directly, e.g. extraction of a tooth, indirectly, e.g. by antibiotics
    b) Ensure good general health.

21. a) Repair when cause is removed or overcome
    b) Suppuration - formation of pus
    c) Extension into adjacent tissues, more rarely to a much wider area
    d) May become chronic.

22. Plasma - to dilute the cause and to carry antibodies and antitoxins to the site.
    White cells - to attack and try to destroy the cause.

23. The reaction of the body to a longstanding injury; often a "walling off" type of tissue response.

24. An abnormal cavity in the body. This cavity is lined and usually has semi-solid or fluid contents.

25. Cell death.

26. An abnormal growth of tissue, serving no useful purpose, and which continues to grow at the expense of the surrounding tissues.

27. Benign - slow growing, localised, harmless.
    Malignant - fast growing, initially localised, later having widespread metastases, often fatal.

28. a) Increase in size of tissue due to the enlargement of cells
    b) Increase in size of tissue due to the increased number of cells
    c) Reduction in size of tissue due to the reduction in cell size or to a decreased number of cells.

<u>Sterilisation</u>

1. Clean off all debris before sterilising.

2. a) Many are poisons
   b) The length of time required
   c) They are not fully effective.

3. By the usual methods e.g. in an autoclave.

4. a) Contaminants may prevent true sterilisation
   b) Contaminants may be more difficult to remove after sterilisation.

5. Autoclave or dry heat.

6. a) Direct heat
   b) Dry heat at too high a temperature.

7. a) Gamma radiation b) Ethylene oxide.

8. Continuous boiling for 29 hours.

9. They may become brittle.

10. a) Steam at high pressure is dangerous
    b) The cycle will have to start again to be completed.

11. a) Packing in suitable bags or boxes
    b) Storing in a suitable antiseptic with rust inhibitor.

12. To avoid infection of the Dental Surgeon and D.A.

13. To prevent their re-use and so reduce the risk of drug addicts getting serum hepatitis.

<u>Preventive Dentistry</u>

1. a) Plaque
   b) Calculus
   c) Poorly finished restorations
   d) Poorly aligned teeth
   e) Ill-fitting dentures or orthodontic appliances.

2. a) Carbohydrate diet
   b) Plaque leading to acid formation
   c) Poor tooth shape and structure.

3. By the action of the tongue, lip and cheeks, and saliva.

4. a) Mucin
   b) Bacteria
   c) Food debris
   d) Dead cells.

5. a) Acids b) Toxins.

6. To assist in the normal formation of bones and teeth.

7. Some of the fluoride is absorbed into the outer enamel surface which makes it more resistant to acid attack.

8. a) In the water supply c) In milk
   b) Fluoride tablets and drops d) In salt (Switzerland).

9. The developing teeth could become mottled.

10. Adequate calcium and vitamins A. and D. in the diet and optimum fluoride intake during the formation of teeth.

11. a) Removal of plaque b) Gum and tongue stimulation.

12. a) Size - not too large for easy use in the mouth
    b) Texture - medium or soft nylon or bristle, unless advised otherwise by Dental Surgeon. Multi-tufted
    c) Shape - straight handle - flat brushing surface.

13. a) Eat fibrous foods at the end of a meal
    b) Vigorous mouth rinsing or use of "Water-pik"
    c) Use of tongue and cheeks
    d) Use of dental floss
    e) Use of wood points
    f) Use of chemical agents e.g. sodium bicarbonate.

14. Detergent - removal of animal and vegetable fats and oils.
    Abrasives - to remove stains.
    Alkaline - to help to neutralise plaque acids.

15. So that a minimal amount of plaque is left on the teeth overnight. During sleep a) salivary flow is reduced so that oral acids are less diluted b) plaque remains undisturbed thus there can be prolonged attack on dental tissues.

16. After using a disclosing solution or tablet, residual plaque will be stained red or blue.

17. After checking for possible hormonal or medical causes; to continue to brush, but carefully and thoroughly, and using the correct textured toothbrush and correct method. Gingivitis is due to plaque.

18. a) Fissure sealants
    b) Prophylactic occlusal fissure amalgams
    c) Topical fluoride.

<u>Periodontics</u>

1. 1 - 2mm.

2. Due to the inflammatory process there is an increased vascular supply.

3. Inflammation of the periodontal membrane.

4. By very good oral hygiene, including inter-dental cleaning.

5. At the gingival margin, as gingivitis.

6. a) Increased plaque and calculus
   b) Greater chance of periodontal disease
   c) Over-eruption of the tooth.

7. a) Drifting of teeth on either side. This leads to loss of contact points and to pocketing
   b) Over-eruption of the opposing tooth. This can lead to pocketing
   c) Increased usage of other teeth, e.g. using the other side of the mouth.

8. Gingivae, periodontal membrane, alveolar bone.

9. Calcified plaque, mainly calcium salts and magnesium.

10. Sub-gingival and supra-gingival.

11. Gingivae, cementum, dentine.

12. This causes least damage to dental tissues. It helps the toothbrush bristles to get between the teeth as far as they can. There is an entirely different method called Bass technique.

13. Mouth breathing predisposes to gingival inflammation.

14. a) Vitamin C is necessary
    b) Fibrous foods have a massaging effect.

15. Aspirin, Phenytoin (used in epilepsy), tobacco, some alkaline toothpastes.

16. Lingual to lower incisors and buccal to upper 6s.

17. Saliva ducts are adjacent to these areas.

18. Mineral salts come from saliva.

19. Blood breakdown products are incorporated into the forming calculus.

20. There is stagnation in the deepening periodontal pocket.

21. The inter-dental papillae. They become ulcerated and appear saucer-shaped.

22. a) Swollen gums
    b) Gums bleed easily
    c) Grey dead tissue on gum surface
    d) Foul smell
    e) Pain
    f) Ulcerated inter-dental papillae
    g) Temperature sometimes raised and glands enlarged.

23. a) Take Metronidazole tablets or antibiotics
    b) Frequent oxygen-releasing antiseptic mouth washes
    c) Very gentle but thorough tooth brushing.

24. Periodontal surgery is carried out to eliminate intra-alveolar "pockets"; whereas a gingivectomy will only eliminate gingival "pockets".

25. Zinc oxide, eugenol and wisps of cotton wool - commercial variations are also available.

26. An abcess involving the periodontal membrane and tissues adjacent to the tooth. Abscess often points lateral to tooth.

27. There is infection and destruction of the periodontal membrane. As the infected area approaches the tooth apex drainage becomes more difficult and an abscess is more likely to develop.

<u>Caries</u>

1. The demineralisation and disintegration of hard tooth substance by acids produced by bacteria.

2. a) Pits and fissures
   b) Interproximal surfaces
   c) The gingival region of a tooth crown
   d) Edges of defective fillings

   These are stagnation areas where plaque collects.

3. a) Visually without aids, i.e. an actual hole, or change in tooth colour
   b) Using mirror and probe
   c) Bite wing radiographs
   d) Transillumination.

4. In stagnation areas such as interstitially, in fissures and at gingival margins. Also around defective restorations and where there is crowding.

5. Due to the cleansing action of the tongue.

6. It contains the bacteria and carbohydrates, which will form acids.

7. It helps to reduce the incidence of caries by washing away food debris. As it is slightly alkaline, it helps to neutralise acids in the mouth.

8. By a white opaque area.

9. During the primary stage of the acid-etch techniques.

10. The roughened surface allows plaque and food debris to collect more easily.

11. Dentine caries can progress rapidly within the enamel shell and without necessarily involving further enamel caries.

12. The layer of sound dentine is getting thin, so that there is easy conduction of heat through the tooth.

13. By laying down secondary dentine in the pulp chamber.

14. The inflammatory exudate increases the pressure in the pulp which stimulates the pulp nerve endings.

15. a) Trauma
    b) Chronic irritation, e.g. by caries or unlined fillings.

16. a) May become chronic, with few symptoms, either as an apical granuloma or as a radicular cyst
    b) May develop into an acute alveolar abscess, and in some cases discharge into the mouth.

17. The opening of a discharging abscess - usually on the outer gum surface and adjacent to a tooth apex.

18. The tooth crown shape is less favourable to stagnation and plaque. These teeth are easy for a patient to clean, and to see that they have been cleaned properly. The tongue and lower lip help in cleansing these teeth. There is usually plenty of saliva in this region to help cleanse the teeth.

19. The tooth substance is more resistant to acid attack. Dental caries in children can be reduced by up to 50%.

20. Attrition is the wearing away of tooth substance by other teeth. Abrasion is the wearing away of tooth substance by external agents, e.g. a toothbrush. Erosion is the loss of tooth substance by chemicals, e.g. acid fruit juices.

Conservative Dentistry

1. a) Restoration of function
   b) Prevention of pain
   c) Restoration of appearance
   d) Maintenance of a healthy pulp
   e) Prevention of further decay.

2. a) The size of the cavity
   b) The amount of tooth crown remaining
   c) The position of the cavity in the tooth and in the mouth.

3. Enamel is a very hard substance and is not easy to cut with a conventional handpiece.

4. There is a microscopic space between the tooth and the restoration into which fluids and micro organisms may pass. Corrosion of the restoration occurs which may show as a discolouration. The amalgam corrosion products form a seal in the microspace and helps to reduce further micro-leakage.

5. They would blunt too quickly.

6. a) The elimination of existing decay
   b) The elimination of stagnation areas to reduce the reoccurrence of decay
   c) The retention of the restoration
   d) The strength of the restoration.

7. By use of a saliva ejector or aspirator and cotton wool rolls or by use of a rubber dam and saliva ejector.

8. a) Assist in condensation of the filling material
   b) To help shape the filling to the tooth and cavity shape
   c) To ensure that the filling gets maximum retention from the cavity's shape
   d) To produce a gloss finish
   e) To reduce the amount of excess filling at the edges of the restoration.

9. a) To relieve or prevent pain
   b) To prevent food lodging in a cavity
   c) To prevent gingival overgrowth.

10. a) They encourage the formation of secondary dentine
    b) They are alkaline and retard the carious process.

11. Protection against thermal and chemical irritation.

12. a) Rubber finger stall
    b) Mortar and pestle
    c) Electric vibrator mixing.

13. The amalgam is weaker. It is more likely that the restoration will break or that the edges will break away.

14. a) By saliva during packing
    b) By hand perspiration if it is handled.

15. There will be excessive expansion resulting in a protruding restoration. Secondary caries may start at these overhanging margins.

16. If there is undue delay, the final amalgam will be weaker (a five minute delay could make it 40% weaker).

17. The D.A. may absorb mercury through the skin, and may develop mercury poisoning.

18. a) To get it to the correct level for occlusion
    b) To shape it for correct masticating function.

19. a) To adapt it to the cavity shape
    b) To reduce the amount of mercury in the filling, and so increase the proportion of silver in the restoration
    c) To reduce air spaces to a minimum.

20. Usually about two hours, but it does vary with different amalgams.

21. Smoothed where possible with stones, finishing burs or sandpaper discs. Interproximally with finishing strips. Finally, polished with paste on a brush or rubber cup or using a special polishing cup or point.

22. a) Improved aesthetics
    b) Better marginal adaptation
    c) Reduced plaque adherence by removing rough and overhanging edges
    d) Production of a smooth surface which reduces corrosion
    e) Elimination of any defects in the surface of the filling.

23. A finishing bur has many more blades so that it smooths rather than cuts.

24. a) It is able to withstand the large masticatory forces
    b) Appearance does not matter.

25. To reduce the risk of mercury vaporisation.

26. a) To prevent absorption of mercury via the skin
    b) To prevent contamination of amalgam by hand moisture and grease.

27. a) As a temporary filling
    b) As a lining for deep cavities.

28. An amalgam cavity has undercuts to help retain the filling. An inlay cavity has no undercuts. This allows the impression of the cavity to be taken and the inlay to be fitted into the cavity.

29. a) To reduce the risk of fracture of a filling due to its size or a heavy bite
b) Because the restoration is part of some complex dentistry - e.g. a bridge
c) To reduce the risk of fracture of the remaining tooth substance by protecting it from occlusal stress.

30. In the indirect technique a model is made from the impression of the tooth and inlay cavity. The gold restoration is made to fit the model. In the direct technique the impression of the cavity is taken in special wax and cast in metal without any other intermediate stages.

31. a) Brown stick composition in a copper ring
b) Rubber base
c) Silicone material.

32. To retract gum from the margin of the prepared tooth and to reduce bleeding.

33. Edge fitting, contacts with adjacent teeth, occlusion with opposing teeth.

34. To ensure perfect adaptation to the tooth so reducing micro-leakage.

35. Zinc phosphate. Zinc polycarboxylate.

36. To a thin creamy consistency.

37. a) To keep the cavity moisture-free
b) To isolate the tooth and retract the gingivae
c) To prevent any material or instruments dropping into the pharynx.

38. Gold and porcelain.

39. From finely ground silica glass.

40. Phosphoric acid and distilled water.

41. To avoid absorption of moisture due to variations in air humidity.

42. Contamination by use of stainless steel instruments during mixing or placement.

43. 21°C.

44. a) The material is brittle and slightly soluble in oral fluids
    b) The material is acid and will damage the pulp if there is any lining deficiency.

45. a) To prevent moisture absorption
    b) To prevent drying out.

46. The material becomes weak and crumbles.

47. To prevent pulpal irritation by the chemicals in the filling material.

48. Mixing silicate and glass ionomer materials. To avoid discolouration of the filling material.

49. a) They are almost insoluble in oral fluids
    b) They are very hard and resistant to wear
    c) Their properties of expansion and contraction are similar to those of teeth
    d) Good colour matching
    e) They can be placed using acid etch techniques.

50. Glass particles in a plastic resin.

51. By the use of a lower proportion of catalyst.

52. a) To fill small interstitial and cervical cavities
    b) They are able to adhere to suitably prepared dentine.

53. By wearing mouth guards.

Paedodontics

1. a) To give the parents dental preventive advice
   b) Treatment, if any, is likely to be simple and should encourage patient co-operation
   c) To allow the child to become familiar with the Dentist, the staff and the equipment.

2. a) Correct toothbrushing
   b) Frequency of toothbrushing
   c) Use of fluoride toothpaste
   d) Use of fluoride tablets
   e) Diet.

3. a) 1) Six week intra-uterine
      2) At birth
      3) At birth
      4) Four years

   b) 1) Six months
      2) Six years
      3) Six years
      4) Ten years.

4. Each layer is thinner in deciduous teeth. Enamel is whiter.

5. a) To keep space for secondary teeth
   b) For masticatory function
   c) To aid speech
   d) To reduce the possibility of the patient getting toothache
   e) To avoid any unpleasant experience of extraction.

6. The root is not fully formed, and the canal will have a wide open apex.

7. A method of killing the pulp of a tooth by sealing certain chemicals in contact with a vital pulp.

8. Because of difficult access to its curved root canals.

9. The tooth will be sensitive to thermal changes.

10. The blood vessels are ruptured by the blow, and the blood in the pulp chamber is slowly decomposed and discolours the dentine.

11. Removal of the pulp tissue in the crown of a tooth. Local anaesthesia is necessary.

12. a) Visual - to observe tooth malposition or fractures or chipping of tooth crown and any soft tissue damage
    b) Palpation - to detect mobility
    c) Electrical or thermal - to check vitality of the tooth
    d) Radiograph - to detect tooth displacement or root fracture.

13. Premature loss of deciduous teeth can lead to loss of space for permanent teeth. Prolonged retention can cause irregularities in the permanent dentition.

14. a) It can improve appearance and reduce the risk of damage to prominent anterior teeth
    b) There is a tendency for treatment to reduce the incidence of caries and periodontal disease
    c) To align teeth prior to restorative procedures.

Crowns and Bridges

1. An artificial replacement covering a large loss of tooth substance.

2. a) Root filling   b) Post crown.

3. To give adequate thickness of the artificial crown for aesthetics, for strength and to allow natural contour of tooth to be reproduced.

4. a) Copper ring and brown stick composition, or
   b) Rubber base or silicone or polyether types, or
   c) Reversible hydrocolloid.

5. Crown scissors.

6. a) Overall impression - to show relationship of the crown to the adjacent teeth
   b) Impression of opposing teeth - to ensure no interference with the bite
   c) Tooth shade - porcelain and acrylic crowns.

7. a) To improve the accuracy of the impression at the neck of the tooth
   b) To reduce bleeding
   c) To retract the gum.

8. a) A tender tooth
   b) A broken crown
   c) Excess wear of the crown
   d) Pain in tempero-mandibular joint
   e) A bite of convenience.

9. a) To protect the tooth from irritation, e.g. thermal changes
   b) Appearance
   c) Prevention of movement, e.g. over-eruption or drifting.

10. a) An artificial replacement for a missing tooth, or teeth which is supported by other teeth and is usually not removable
    b) Abutments and pontic.

11. Gold, porcelain. Acrylic facings can be used.

12. Caries rate; periodontal condition; the occlusion; roots of the abutment teeth; size of the bridge.

13. They are firmly held in place. They are usually about the same size as the natural teeth, so they cause less interference with speech etc. They prevent movement of the adjacent teeth.

14. Dental cements e.g. zinc oxyphosphate, polycarboxylate.

15. Usually more than one crown is involved, so that plenty of time may be required. The fit of crowns is very close, so that any excess cement must be able to squeeze out so that the bridge is seated properly.

<u>Endodontics</u>

1. "Endo" meaning "in" therefore - inside tooth treatment. This will include all forms of pulp therapy - mummification, pulpotomy, pulpectomy, etc.

2. To render the tooth free from pain and infection. This will in turn prevent further infection of the periapical area from the root canal.

3. To show the root canal's shape and length and to show any possible obstruction or any periapical infection.

4. a) 1
   b) 2
   c) 3
   d) 1
   e) 1
   f) 3

5. Irritation due to chemical and thermal changes, to trauma. Infection, e.g. caries.

6. The pulp contains numerous nerve fibres most of which may be dead in an infected pulp but some nerve fibres could still be alive.

7. Non vital pulp - usually due to caries.

8. The inflammatory exudate causes pressure on nerve endings in the periodontal membrane.

9. a) Dry heat at 140°C for three hours, or 160°C for one hour
   b) Chemical disinfectants.

10. Dry heat at 160°C for one hour.

11. a) Disinfectants
    b) Antibiotics.

12. To assist in the removal of debris and disinfection of the root canal. To help to kill micro-organisms.

13. When a rubber dam is not being used.

14. a) Elimination of caries, removal of pulp debris and irrigation
    b) Reaming
    c) Sterilisation
    d) Drying
    e) Filling.

15. a) To reduce risk of contamination of the root canal by oral bacteria
    b) To keep the teeth dry
    c) To prevent inhalation or swallowing of instruments, etc.

16. By the use of cotton wool rolls and adequate suction.

17. Finding and exploring root canals. They are used with radiographs to measure the length of a root canal.

18. Engine - rotary and giromatic. Hand.

19. a) To clean, straighten and shape the root canal
    b) To smooth walls of the root canal
    c) Used in the slow running handpiece to carry root filling paste up the root canal.

20. To ensure a good fit of the gutta percha or silver point.

21. It oscillates through a right angle only.

22. a) The small ones are flexible so that they will adapt to curved canals
    b) They are less likely to fracture than other types of reamer.

23. a) The range of sizes is limited
    b) They do not produce a tapered canal to fit gutta percha or silver points.

24. a) To absorb pus and blood from the canal
    b) To help to dry the canal
    c) To carry medicaments into the canal.

25. To kill micro-organisms in the root canal.

26. Yes.

27. No.

28. By measurements obtained from a diagnostic radiograph taken with a measuring instrument in the root canal.

29. To help form a complete apical seal by filling accessory canals and any discrepancy between the point and the root canal.

30. a) To form, with root sealer paste, a complete seal of the main apical foramen
    b) To help to push root sealer paste into lateral root canals.

31. It is easier to prepare the root canal for a post crown.

32. a) With very fine canals
    b) In curved root canals.

33. a) Drainage through the root canal
    b) Incision of the gum.

34. a) Frequent hot salt water mouth washes
    b) Full oral hygiene.

35. a) Following trauma
b) In a small number of cases in crown and bridge work - usually when a tooth is in a slightly abnormal position.

36. The surgical removal of the apex of a tooth.

37. An amalgam restoration placed at the root apex during an apicectomy. Used to ensure a good apical seal.

Physiology

1. The study of the functions of normal body systems.

2. Food and oxygen.

3. a) Basic metabolism b) Activity.

4. Lungs, kidneys, skin and to a lesser extent, the liver.

5. External respiration - the exchange of gases (O_2 and CO_2) between the lungs and the environment.
Internal respiration - the exchange of gases (O_2 and CO_2) between cells and their fluid environment.

6. Nose, nasopharynx, larynx, trachea, bronchi, bronchioles, alveolar ducts, alveoli, alveolar membrane, capillary wall, capillary.

7. a) To remove any airway obstruction
b) To increase and decrease the volume of the thoracic cavity, thus encouraging the movement of air into and out of the lungs.

8. Exercise, fear, excitement.

9. Attached to the haemoglobin in the red cells.

10. Mainly dissolved in plasma. Some is attached to the haemoglobin in the red cells.

11. The heart, arteries, arterioles, capillaries, venules, veins.

12. The pressure wave set up in the blood stream when the heart pumps more blood into the arteries.

13. Right atrium - collection of blood from the tissues.
Right ventricle - pumps blood via pulmonary arteries to the lungs.
Left atrium - receives blood from the pulmonary veins.
Left ventricle - pumps blood via the aorta and arterial system to the tissues.

14. To allow blood to flow in one direction only.

15. Oxygenated blood.

16. Via the coronary arteries.

17. Fibrin, platelets, red and white blood cells.

18. a) To prevent excessive loss of blood
    b) To start the wound repair process.

19. When damaged they produce thromboplastin which helps to produce the fibrin framework of the blood clot. Platelets lodge in this framework and help to build up the clot.

20. 5 litres (70ml per Kg body weight).

21. 70mls.

22. Low haemoglobin content of blood.

23. Plasma - 55% (90% of which is water)
    Cells - 45% (Red cells 5 million per cubic millimetre
    White cells 8,000 per cubic millimetre
    Platelets 250,000 per cubic millimetre).

24. They are part of the defence mechanism of the body.

25. To filter off micro-organisms and foreign bodies. To manufacture lymphocytes.

26. a) To collect tissue fluids from tissues and to return them to the blood stream
    b) To collect excretory products from the cells
    c) To produce certain white cells
    d) To transport fat from the small intestine.

27. Complex food molecules need to be broken down into smaller absorbable and useful molecules. Insoluble substances need to be converted into soluble substances.

28. Carbohydrates (starch and sugars), fats, proteins, mineral salts, water, vitamins and roughage.

29. In the mouth.

30. Biting and chewing of the food mixes it with saliva. The saliva contains the enzyme ptyalin or amylase which starts the digestion of starches.

31. a) The nasal cavity is protected by the soft palate and posterior pharyngeal wall
    b) The larynx is protected by the closure of the epiglottis.

32. a) To mix food particles with saliva
    b) To keep food between the teeth.

33. a) To produce a large surface area for the action of enzymes
    b) To produce pieces of food of a reasonable size for swallowing.

34. An organic catalyst which speeds the rate of digestion.

35. Adequate - enough for energy and growth needs.
    Balanced - all the essential constituents should be present in correct proportions.

36. Age, sex, type of activity performed, e.g. occupation.

37. Frequently as long as three hours, sometimes even longer.

38. To lubricate the food and to protect the walls of the alimentary canal.

39. a) To kill many micro-organisms
    b) Gastric enzymes need an acid medium
    c) To stop the action of amylase.

40. Simple molecule foods, e.g. glucose, alcohol.

41. a) Absorption of end products of digestion
    b) Water absorption.

42. These are chemical senses and therefore need the odour or flavour to be in solution to stimulate the sensory nerve endings.

43. On the upper (dorsal) surface of the tongue.

44. a) The protection of internal and external body surfaces
    b) There are special types of epithelium, e.g. secretory
    c) Prevention of excessive loss of body fluids
    d) Temperature maintenance.

45. a) To give body shape and support
    b) To provide attachments for muscles
    c) Protection of vital organs, e.g. brain, heart.

46. a) Osteoclasts are bone dissolving cells
    b) Osteoblasts are bone forming cells.

First Aid

1. To prevent adverse reactions and emergencies. To carry out treatment knowing the possible problems which might occur.

2. a) Floors - by reporting loose mats, slippery or uneven surfaces
   b) Electrical - by reporting loose wires and inadequate lighting
   c) Furniture - by reporting weak legs, projections, etc.

3. a) Careful suction and guarding of the cheeks and tongue
   b) By making protective goggles available to the patient
   c) By making sure instruments are cool
   d) By not passing instruments or materials across the patient's face.

4. Fainting and shock, asphyxia, diabetes, heart and kidney diseases, poisoning.

5. Sudden and severe drop in blood pressure.

6. Nausea, vomiting, fainting.

7. Pallor, sweating, rapid, weak pulse, lowered level of consciousness.

8. Primary shock - fear, alarm, temper.
   Secondary shock - prolonged or severe loss of blood.

9. Lay him/her down, keep him/her warm but not over-heated.

10. Loss of blood pressure, of red cells, of white cells and shortage of oxygen, cardiac arrest, death.

11. Apply pressure to the wound to stop the bleeding; get the patient to rest. Summon help.

12. Epilepsy, hysteria. There are other less common reasons.

13. A burn is caused by dry heat, a scald by wet heat.

14. a) Remove the cause
    b) Prevent or treat shock
    c) Cover with a sterile dressing which has been wetted with sterile cold water.

15. a) Switch off electricity supply.
    b) Apply artificial respiration if necessary
    c) Treat as for burns.

16. Patient has a warning - aura. Loss of consciousness sometimes with alternate muscle contraction and relaxation. Incontinence.

17. a) Prevent him from injuring himself by removing obvious danger, e.g. electric fire
    b) Protect tongue, if possible use nothing hard
    c) Place in the tonsillar position
    d) Maintain airway.

18. The patient appears distressed, pale, sweaty and cold, dizzy and nauseated and may lose consciousness. The pulse is rapid and weak.

19. The fetus may press on the inferior vena cava and restrict the return of blood to the heart.

20. a) If possible immobilise the part
    b) Get patient to hospital - probably by ambulance.

<u>Drugs</u>

1. a) Relief of pain
   b) Sleep induction
   c) Promotion of a feeling of well-being
   d) Encourages sleep.

2. Aspirin can be very irritant, therefore aspirin tablets should not be sucked, nor taken on an empty stomach. Soluble forms are preferable. Aspirin is contra-indicated in some medical conditions.

3. Antiseptic - a chemical which prevents the growth of bacteria (bacteriostasis) and which may kill some bacteria (bacteriocidal).
   Antibiotic - a biological substance which kills or inhibits the growth of certain micro-organisms.

4. Prophylactic drug therapy.

5. To reduce the risk of blood clotting in blood vessels. Associated with cardio-vascular disease.

6. a) The patient may be allergic to the drug
   b) Sometimes gastro-intestinal upsets occur
   c) Some micro-organisms become resistant.

7. Where there is a history of rheumatic heart disease, heart murmurs or if the patient has ever undergone cardiac surgery.

8. a) To allay fear
   b) To reduce secretions
   c) To make the patient more co-operative
   d) To facilitate a smooth anaesthetic.

9. Usually orally or intravenously. Diazepam. Pentobarbitone. Atropine.

10. In the treatment of medical conditions such as rheumatoid arthritis and asthma.

11. They suppress inflammatory response. An unwanted side effect is to reduce the natural production of cortico steroids. This will reduce the patient's ability to withstand stress, and they are more likely to collapse.

12. It indicates that the patient is taking certain psychiatric drugs and might mean that local anaesthetics containing adrenalin should only be used with care.

13. a) Identify the poison if possible
    b) Give specific or general antidote if the poison is corrosive
    c) If the poison is non-corrosive, encourage vomiting
    d) Get medical assistance.

14. A substance which kills fungi. Nystatin or Amphotericin B used in the treatment of denture sore mouth.

15. A chemical which kills tissue and prevents the growth of organisms.

<u>Local Anaesthesia</u>

1. a) Elimination of pain
   b) Control of haemorrhage
   c) As an aid to diagnosis.

2. a) Local infiltration
   b) Regional or block anaesthesia
   c) Surface anaesthesia.

3. The injection of local anaesthetic solution into the medullary bone.

4. It blocks nerve impulses along the sensory pathway.

5. Infection may be spread by the procedure. Local anaesthetics are less efficient in the presence of inflammation.

6. a) Anaesthesia of the mucous membrane to aid the painless insertion of a local anaesthetic syringe needle
   b) An aid to the removal of very loose deciduous teeth
   c) For deep scaling
   d) For minor procedures involving gingivae.

7. a) Industrially, usually by irradiation then the cartridge is placed in a sealed pack.
   b) By keeping it immersed in antiseptic solution
   c) By flaming. This will kill some micro-organisms.

8. a) Anaesthetic agent
   b) Usually a vaso-constrictor
   c) An antiseptic
   d) A preservative
   e) Isotonic water for injection.

9. a) They are always sharp
   b) They are very thin, therefore easier penetration is obtained
   c) They are already sterile
   d) They reduce the risk of transmitting serum hepatitis.

10. To reduce pain during the injection of the solution.

11. Test the syringe to
   a) Check that the needle is unblocked
   b) Expel air from the cartridge.

12. The taste of the solution is very bitter.

13. a) Cartridge - long $1\frac{5}{8}$" - short 1". Usually gauge 27.
   b) Hypodermic - gauges 1 to 27 - various lengths.

14. Inferior dental and lingual nerves - sometimes the long buccal as well.

15. a) To restrict the diffusion of local anaesthetic solution, which will
      1) Prolong the period of analgesia
      2) Ensure a high level of analgesia
   b) The haemostatic effect is sometimes useful in surgery.

16. It allows the Dental Surgeon to check that he is not injecting into a blood vessel.

17. It may cause the patient to faint.

18. Fainting, due to nervousness.

19. a) The needle may be unsterile
   b) The needle may break
   c) The needle will damage soft tissues but may also damage a nerve or blood vessel.

20. The cartridge could be contaminated and lead to cross infection.

21. Partial loss of nerve sensation.

22. Injury to, or pressure on a nerve. This may be due to direct physical injury or to inflammatory change.

23. A blood vessel in a muscle may have been damaged by the needle leading to bleeding and fibrosis.

<u>Extractions and Minor Oral Surgery</u>

1. Caries. Periodontal disease.

2. a) 2
   b) 3
   c) 1
   d) 1
   e) 2
   f) 3
   g) 2.

3. a) No rinsing for 24 hours
   b) No exercise
   c) No alcohol
   d) No hot fluids
   e) No smoking.

4. A blood clot forms to fill the socket. This clot becomes organised initially as granulation tissue then forming fibrous tissue and new capillaries, later bone is formed. Epithelium grows across the surface.

5. Where there is little or no blood clot in a tooth socket - the bony socket walls become exposed and frequently become infected.

6. There is virtually no blood clot so that healing takes plac from the bone surfaces.

7. To lift soft tissue away from underlying bone. It is sometimes used to retract tissue and to protect tissues whe using cutting instruments.

8. Toothed tissue forceps.

9. Rinsing might dislodge the forming blood clot and raised blood pressure might lead to continuous slow bleeding.

10. a) To help keep the socket clean and free from food.
    b) To encourage vaso-dilation, and hence the healing process.

    N.B. Salt is a mild antiseptic. Wait 24 hours until the clot is well formed, and so unlikely to lead to further bleeding.

11. Suture pack containing needle holder, tissue forceps, scissors, cheek retractor and sucker.

12. Curved cutting needles. Black silk thread or resorbable catgut.

13. a) The edges of the wound will have started to heal
    b) There is little risk of bleeding.
    c) The sutures become loose and irritate the patient.
    d) They are foreign bodies and an acute inflammatory reaction will occur in the tissues.

14. a) Removing sterile instruments from a steriliser
    b) Removing sterile instruments from their packs when laying up trays and trolleys.

15. a) By explaining in simple terms what is going to happen
    b) By remaining calm herself, and by reassuring the patient
    c) By not displaying instruments.

16. A procedure in which there is planned cutting of the oral mucosa.

17. a) Removal of buried teeth, roots or impacted teeth
    b) Periodontal surgery
    c) Repair of oro-antral fistula.
    d) Biopsy
    e) Apicectomy
    f) Removal of cysts.

18. Surgical removal of the apex of a tooth.

19. The surgical removal of a piece of tissue for examination under a microscope, after preparation by cutting sections and staining.

20. Place the tissue in formal saline solution to send for pathological investigation.

21. a) To retract cheeks, tongue and soft tissues at the site of operation
    b) Elevation of roots or teeth requiring light forces
    c) Elevation of roots or teeth requiring medium forces.

22. One which cannot erupt into normal position due to obstruction by another tooth, or by bone.

23. a) Disto-angular
    b) Mesio-angular
    c) Horizontal
    d) Vertical.

24. a) Pericoronitis
    b) Caries
    c) Apical abscess.

25. a) Adequate room for access and visibility to the underlying tissues
    b) Avoidance of important nerves and blood vessels
    c) A good blood supply to ensure healing.

26. In the limited room available, a curved needle makes it easier to pass through the tissues.

27. Infection introduced into the wound would delay healing, cause the patient discomfort and retard recovery.

28. Acute or chronic inflammation of bone.

29. Lingual nerve.

30. An abnormal connection between the maxillary antrum and the mouth.

31. The roots of the upper premolars and molars lie immediately below the antrum - sometimes some of the bone forming the floor of the antrum is extracted with the tooth.

32. When the Dental Surgeon considers that the extraction of a tooth may have created a fistula, the patient should be advised not to blow his nose, or rinse vigorously for a few days.

33. The track along which an abscess has discharged to the surface.

34. Caries.

35. The removal of tooth supporting bone. To prepare the mouth for dentures. To improve a patient's appearance.

36. Inflammation in the soft tissues around the crown of a tooth.

37. It is often associated with partially erupted lower wisdom teeth. Food stagnates under the gum flap and gives rise to inflammation, which may be acute or chronic.

38. To reduce contamination of the wound.

39. Coupland's chisel, mallet and bone chisel, Rongeurs bone nibblers, burs, bone files.

40. To syringe sockets with sterile water or saline solution.

41. Blades are blunted in use, so each patient has a sharp blade. Reduces the incidence of cross infection.

42. a) As elevators b) Removal of bone.

43. Coagulation of blood at the site of a damaged blood vessel.

44. Immediately a blood vessel is damaged.

45. 1 - 6 hours after extraction.

46. When the vasoconstrictor effect of the local anaesthetic wears off there is vasodilatation. The inflammatory response to tissue injury is also occurring. These together can lead to further haemorrhage.

47. a) Remove excess blood clot with the aid of a clean gauze
    b) Roll up gauze swabs to thick finger size
    c) Place over socket
    d) Get patient to bite on this pack for at least five minutes
    e) Repeat if necessary
    f) If bleeding persists call Dental Surgeon
    g) Record on patient's notes. In any case, report what you have done to the Dental Surgeon.

48. From the fourth day after extraction and onwards.

49. Infection in the wound leading to breakdown of the healing blood vessels.

General Disease

1. Inflammation.

2. Patients complain of their symptoms; doctors and dentists detect signs.

3. An organism which, under normal circumstances, does not cause disease.

4. The virulence of the organism and the resistance of the body.

5. By the blood stream; by the lymph; through adjacent tissues.

6. A collection of pus consisting of inflammatory exudate, tissue debris, leucocytes and micro-organisms; contained within a cavity lined by a pyogenic membrane.

7. An increase in the body temperature due to disease.

8. Acute and chronic. In the acute form the cause is too severe for the immediate body defence to overcome. In the chronic form there is a slow smouldering reaction in which tissue repair and destruction occur simultaneously.

9. A non-traumatic break in a body surface.

10. Additional bacteria may get into the blood stream, and might cause further damage in an already damaged heart.

11. A male with an hereditory bleeding disorder.

UNIVERSITY COLLEGE CORK Library

12. The abnormal loss of blood from a blood vessel.

13. Blood clotting.

14. An abnormal blood clot occurring within a blood vessel.

15. Fragments of the thrombus can become detached - they are known as emboli. They circulate in the blood stream and can block small vessels leading to thrombosis. This will be serious if the heart, brain or lungs are affected.

16. Technically lack of blood supply and oxygen to a part of the brain. Usually caused by a blood clot, a tumour or a haemorrhage.

17. To reduce the danger of blood clots forming in damaged blood vessels.

18. General anaesthesia is usually contra-indicated, as are local anaesthetics containing adrenaline. The anti-coagulant drug may need to be adjusted by the doctor to prevent excessive haemorrhage.

19. Inflammation of the bronchial tubes.

20. Air pollution, cigarette smoking, repeated attacks of acute bronchitis, chronic infection of the nasal sinuses.

21. Chronic cough and sputum - worse in the mornings. Breathlessness on exertion.

22. Paralysis associated with damage to cranial nerve VII.

23. There are two forms, but it usually means a condition where there is a lack of insulin, so that the breakdown of sugars and carbohydrates is abnormal.

24. Under the stress of dentistry a diabetic patient may produce a low blood sugar content and feel faint. Give the patient some glucose, and then get him to balance his insulin.

25. a) A
    b) A
    c) C
    d) D
    e) B.

Radiography

1. To reduce radiation hazards.

2. Silver salts in the emulsion surface of the film undergo change when exposed to X-radiation. The developed radiograph is darker with increased dosage of X-rays.

3. The metal absorbs the X-rays, preventing them from getting to the film, and so stops them from causing changes on the film.

4. It is part of the electromagnetic spectrum possessing very short penetrating rays.

5. A fully processed X-ray film.

6. a) Keep away from stray radiation
   b) Keep away from dampness and heat
   c) Keep away from direct sunlight
   d) Keep away from fumes.

7. Placed in a light tight cassette under dark room conditions.

8. a) Density of tissue.
   b) Thickness of overlying tissues
   c) Speed of the film.

9. a) Interproximal and occlusal caries
   b) The state of the bone crests between the teeth.

10. Intensifying screens.

11. To produce a picture of one tooth with the whole of the surrounding tissues.

12. The cheek teeth, i.e. premolars and molars.

13. Maxilla, mandible, the teeth and cervical spine.

14. Skin, nails, hair, blood cells and bone marrow, reproductive organs, eyes.

15. a) Do not hold films for the patient
    b) Do not stand in front of the X-ray tube i.e. the line of the primary beam
    c) Ideally, stand behind a wall or protective screen at least two metres behind and to the side of the tube
    d) Wear a lead apron.

16. a) Regular checking of the apparatus by experts
    b) Unplug the machine when not actually in use
    c) Use a small aperture diaphragm.

17. a) By use of a radiation detector film
    b) By use of specialised detection equipment.

18. a) By shutting herself in the dark room and switching off all lights including the safelight. Within a minute the eyes will be accustomed to the dark and any leakage of light will become obvious
b) Leave an unwrapped film on the bench for 2-3 minutes, then process this film.

19. The glass filter permits the passage of light at a wavelength which will not affect the film during the short time that the film is open in the dark room.

20. Silver halide and gelatin.

21. a) See that the patient's name has been recorded on the film hanger
b) Check that the dark room is light proof
c) Tear the envelope carefully
d) Take care not to discard the film
e) Handle the film with care e.g. avoid fingerprints on the film
f) Do not unduly delay getting the film into the developer.

22. a) Check the patients' names are with the radiographs
b) Check the temperature and volume of the developing and fixing solutions
c) Check the timer is available
d) Check that the safelight is working
e) Check the availability of film hangers.

23. a) To dislodge any surface air bubbles
b) To ensure that even development takes place.

24. To reduce the chance of dermatitis, or staining of the clothes.

25. To allow for the full processing of the crystals in the film emulsion.

26. To remove developer agents and so prevent contamination of the fixing solution. This will also prevent the possibility of producing "fogging".

27. a) To dissolve out crystals in the emulsion that have not undergone change, due to exposure. This would lead to discoloration
b) To neutralise chemical reactions on the film
c) To produce a visible image
d) To harden the emulsion on the film.

28. a) Underexposure, underdevelopment
b) Faulty safelight, old film, overexposure to safelight, prolonged development, poor film storage conditions.

29. a) Incorrect positioning of the X-ray tube
    b) Some absorbing object between the X-ray tube and the patient
    c) The film not fully immersed in processing solutions
    d) Contact with another object during developing.

30. If filed damp, the film surface may be damaged.

31. Loose in small envelopes, labelled with the patient's name, the date taken, the area radiographed, or mounted on cellumat on which the patient's name is written and then placed in the envelope.

Orthodontics

1. From the Greek meaning 'straight teeth'.

2. a) The growth and development of teeth, jaws and face
   b) The function of the oral-facial soft tissue.

3. Prevention or correction of irregularities of tooth position.

4. A condition in which the upper and lower teeth do not meet in the normal manner.

5. a) Hereditory, e.g. large teeth and small jaws
   b) Premature loss or prolonged retention of deciduous teeth
   c) Soft tissue behaviour, e.g. tongue thrusting.

6. a) The horizontal overlap between the upper and lower incisal edges
   b) The vertical overlap of the anterior teeth
   c) Insufficient space for the number of teeth present in the jaws.

7. a) Class I - normal occlusion
   b) Class II - where the upper incisor teeth meet anterior to normal occlusion
   c) Class III - the lower teeth meet edge to edge with the upper teeth, or may protrude.

8. a) The patient's notes
   b) Radiographs
   c) Models.

9. Bone is a living tissue and is able to be moulded. The bone is absorbed on one side of the tooth socket, and new bone is laid down on the other side of the socket.

10. a) It creates space near the front of the arches to allow the upper anterior teeth to be retracted
    b) Extractions further back would mean moving more teeth, which takes longer.

11. The Labial Fraenum.

12. Sometimes it is associated with a space between the upper permanent incisors, and is removed to assist closure of the space. Fraenectomy.

13. An appliance which cannot be removed by the patient as it is cemented or bonded to the teeth.

14. a) They are made in the laboratory and so save surgery time
    b) They are easy for the Dental Surgeon to adjust
    c) They are easy for the patient to clean properly
    d) They have some advantages in appearance.

15. a) The patient is able to mishandle them, bending wires or breaking the appliance
    b) The patient can leave them out
    c) There are limitations to the tooth movements which can be carried out e.g. rotations need a fixed appliance.

16. A crib is a stainless steel wire which grips a tooth to help retain an appliance. A labial bow is a stainless steel wire around the labial surface of several anterior teeth, either to help retain the appliance or to move back the anterior teeth. A spring is a stainless steel wire designed to move individual teeth.

17. a) Wear it all the time unless the Dental Surgeon advises otherwise
    b) Keep appointments for adjustment
    c) Clean carefully after all meals
    d) Return to Dental Surgeon immediately if teeth hurt, or the appliance breaks
    e) Do not interfere with the wires on the appliance
    f) Eating and talking may be different for the first 24 hours.

General Anaesthesia

1. Loss of consciousness with loss of ALL sensations.

2. It is produced by drugs administered by inhalation or by injection.

3. Acute inflammation; multiple extractions; major surgery; age (children); mentally and physically handicapped patients; the very nervous patient.

4. a) Nitrous oxide, oxygen and Halothane
   b) Methohexitone, Thiopentone.

5. a) To ensure that they are all present
   b) To check that they are not out of date.

6. a) Emergency kit, e.g. airways laryngoscope, endotracheal tubes. Suitable drugs.
   b) Syringe and needle if intravenous agent is to be used
   c) Mouth prop and gags
   d) Mouth packs
   e) Suitable tips for suction machine
   f) Appropriate dental instruments.

7. In case it is necessary to make contact in an emergency.

8. At each examination and before prescribing drugs.

9. To act as chaperone.

10. The administration of anaesthetic gases by a rubber tube which passes through the nose and larynx into the trachea.

11. It secures the patient's airway. It prevents blood etc. getting into the lungs. It allows better access to the mouth.

12. The vapours diffuse from the alveoli of the lungs into the blood as it passes through the pulmonary blood vessels. This blood is then pumped to the brain.

13. Advantages - accuracy of dosage, speed of onset, no smell, no mask
    Disadvantages - some patients are upset by the thought of injections, great care is required in the calculation of the dosage.

14. It is a colourless, non-inflammable gas, with faint smell and taste; supplied in cylinders. It is a weak narcotic (sleep inducing) but has analgesic properties.

15. 20%. This is necessary to maintain the oxygen level in the blood at approximately normal level; this will ensure adequate oxygen to the brain.

16. Low oxygen i.e. less than atmospheric air.

17. The patient may have a bluish colour to the skin, and there may be convulsions. The patient breathes hard in an effort to obtain sufficient oxygen.

18. It is an inhalation anaesthetic. The N_2O/O_2 gas mixture picks up Halothane vapour as it passes through the Halothane vaporizer.

19. It produces sleep and allows at least 20% oxygen to be used whilst maintaining a smooth anaesthetic.

20. It is supplied as a white powder, and is mixed with sterile water for injection to produce a 1% solution. This solution can be injected into a suitable vein.

21. a) Check the cylinders of oxygen and nitrous oxide, and the Halothane reservoir
    b) Connect the tubes and masks
    c) Turn on cylinders and check the machine is working.

22. a) By efficient pain-reduced treatment
    b) By use of premedication drugs which reduce anxiety.

23. a) Check that the patient has followed pre-operation instructions, especially nil by mouth
    b) Check that the patient has no cough or cold
    c) Ask the patient to go to the toilet
    d) Check that the patient is wearing suitable loose clothing
    e) Check that the patient has signed the consent form
    f) Remove the patient's dentures and glasses if any.

24. a) By doing her best to ensure that the patient is seen on time
    b) By being sympathetic with voice and actions
    c) By explaining what will happen.

25. To reduce the possibility of vomiting.

26. The laryngeal reflex is depressed during a general anaesthetic and vomit could enter the lungs, causing bronchospasm, respiratory obstruction, pneumonia or death.

27. The cords will close to protect the lungs and prevent oxygen from reaching the lungs.

28. The vocal cords are nearly closed and air passing through this restriction causes the crowing noise (called laryngeal stridor). The condition is called laryngospasm.

29. To prevent foreign bodies or saliva entering the larynx.

30. The sense of hearing is the last sense to be lost, and the first to return.

31. It reduces the possibility of fainting. The effect of vasodilatation is reduced thus blood pressure is less likely to fall to a level which reduces oxygenation of the brain.

32. The carotid artery in the neck will usually provide a visible and palpable pulse. The chest movements can be observed, or a hand near the nose will feel the air flow.

33. Into the tonsillar position. This is preferable to horizontal, face up, as it helps to prevent airway obstruction by the tongue, and if the patient vomits there is a reduced chance of inhaling the vomit.

34. a) Respiratory obstruction
    b) Hypotension
    c) Respiratory arrest
    d) Cardiac arrest.

35. The effects of an anaesthetic take about twelve hours to wear off properly so that patients' reactions may be slowed for this length of time.

36. The use of drugs to calm the emotions and as a result, raise the pain threshold. The drugs may be administered orally, intravenously or by inhalation (relative analgesia).

37. The method is very reliable and safe. A small amount of the drug is used. Rapid onset and rapid recovery. Amnesia.

38. Not to drive cars etc. or to use machinery that day. To arrange that the patient is accompanied by a responsible adult. That the patient may remain drowsy for some hours.

39. a) Ensure that the patient can breathe properly
    b) Move patient into tonsillar position preferably with head slightly down
    c) Administer oxygen
    d) Summon help
    e) Diagnose cause of collapse.

40. a) Secure the airway - check that there is no obstruction in the mouth, pharynx or larynx - check that there is no restriction to breathing e.g. tight clothing
    b) After these checks administer oxygen.

41. Deprivation of oxygen can lead to severe brain damage.

42. Pooled in the legs and abdomen.

43. There will be increased venous blood to the heart therefore increased cardiac output and the heart will more easily perfuse the brain with oxygenated blood.

44. External cardiac massage - i.e. application of pressure to the patient's sternum about sixty times per minute.

Materials

1. Conservation - temporary filling) with Eugenol
   - lining)
   - polishing fillings
   Prosthetics - in zinc oxide/Eugenol paste for reline impressions and special tray impressions
   Endodontics - with Eugenol as a root sealer
   Periodontics - with Eugenol and cotton wool as a periodontal pack
   Surgery - with Eugenol and cotton wool as a socket pack.

2. Conservation - linings
   - fixing crowns and inlays
   - temporary filling
   Orthodontics - fixing stainless steel bands to teeth
   Oral surgery - fixing splints to teeth.

3. To match similar minute changes of the teeth.

4. Sheet wax - used in denture work and occlusal registration
   Stick wax - blue for inlay work
   - sticky - e.g. as an impression tray adhesive
   Ribbon wax - used in tray modification and occlusal registration
   Wax patterns - for cast metal denture construction
   Composition - wax is a major constituent.

5. Greenstick composition. Peripheral seal material.

6. a) Powder tin not shaken to mix the contents
   b) Too much powder, caused by tapping the powder scoop
   c) Water too warm
   d) Insufficient spatulation.

7. Indirect technique
   a) Copper ring and brown stick composition or copper ring and rubber base impression material. Both require a full arch impression taken in alginate or rubber base
   b) Full arch rubber base using thin wash for cavity detail
   c) Reversible hydrocolloid. Full opposing arch alginate impression.

   Direct technique - blue inlay wax.

8. a) Preliminary impressions for full dentures
   b) Impressions for mouth splints
   c) Impressions for single inlays or crowns.

9. Place on gauze in a bowl of warm water. When soft it should be moulded by hand and replaced in warm water to ensure that uniform softness is maintained.

10. The material becomes sticky and looses its properties.

11. Root canal fillings; temporary filling material; soft lining for dentures or splints. Testing pulp vitality.

12. a) Full and partial denture occlusal checks
    b) Natural occlusion checks
    c) Crown, bridge and inlay occlusal checks.

13. a) Non-irritant to dentine
    b) Not easily dislodged from the cavity by the patient
    c) Easily removed by the dentist.

14. Epimines e.g. Scutan, Mouth curing acrylics e.g. Trim; composites; silicates; celluloid crown forms; acrylic crown forms cemented with zinc oxide/Eugenol cements.

15. Unfilled resins, e.g. Nuvaseal. Filled resins with acid etch techniques e.g. composites. Amalgam.

16. A mild acid solution is applied to the tooth, cleansing the enamel surface and removing small amounts of enamel (etching) thus creating hundreds of short tubular deficiencies in the enamel surface. The resin fills these tubular deficiencies and when set provides hundreds of anchorage tags. The resin will chemically bond to the appropriate filling material, helping to retain the restoration and reduce micro-leakage.

Prosthetics

1. False eyes, nose, ear, leg, hand.

2. a) Function (eating and speech)
   b) TM joint position
   c) Appearance (lip contour and vertical height).

3. An artificial replacement for one or more teeth and their supporting structures in an arch, but not for all the teeth.

4. Acrylic (methyl methacrylate), cobalt chrome, gold.

5. Impression composition; plaster of Paris; zinc oxide - Eugenol paste; silicone or rubber materials; alginate.

6. a) Retching
   b) Due to materials touching the back of the tongue.

7. Tray perforation; special adhesive; softened sticky wax; sticky wax and cotton wool.

8. A detached impression leads to an inaccurate model.

9. Distortion can begin to occur.

10. An impression of the mouth taking account of the position of the tissues during eating, swallowing and speaking.

11. a) Wash off any debris or saliva
    b) Carefully wrap it in a damp cloth and seal it in a plastic bag bearing the patient's name, at all times taking care not to distort the impression
    c) Get it to the laboratory as soon as possible.

12. It will distort, leading to an inaccurate model, and an ill-fitting denture or appliance.

13. Room temperature.

14. To ensure greater accuracy of the final impression.

15. By tracing the periphery with a special material such as greenstick composition, or one of the mouth setting acrylics or rubber base material.

16. The length and position of all the upper teeth; the vertical distance between the jaws, the naturally retruded position of the mandible, sometimes the protrusive position.

17. Tooth shade, tooth shape and lip contour.

18. As the dentures are in wax it allows easy adjustment to correct any errors of teeth and gumwork or to accommodate changed ideas.

19. The appearance of the dentures; the periphery of the wax dentures; the vertical and horizontal relationships of the jaws. The shade of the teeth.

20. a) Stretched skin around the mouth, as if they had a full mouth
    b) Sunken - especially the lips; and showing folds at the mouth corners.

21. a) By selection of suitably shaped anterior teeth.
    b) By slight variation in the setting of individual teeth, e.g. producing gaps or slight rotations
    c) By showing the correct amount of tooth when the patient is at rest or talking
    d) By giving correct support for the lips and cheeks
    e) By incisal grinding.

22. To form a vacuum and food seal.

23. They should be kept moist as the acrylic base can shrink if it dries out.

24. To indicate errors in occlusion in all movements (high spots).

25. a) Wearing and cleaning instructions
    b) Advice about returning if adjustments are needed
    c) Advice on mouth changes and the need to return for regular examination
    d) To keep dentures moist.

26. There is little suction and the movement of the tongue frequently dislodges the denture.

27. A material used on the fitting surface of a denture which remains soft at mouth temperature for some time. It helps to cushion the mucosa from pressure of the denture.

28. By making a new denture or by relining.

29. Denture hyperplasia.

30. Zinc oxide - Eugenol paste. Some tissue conditioners can also be used.

31. A plastic material which takes a few days to set. It allows the denture bearing tissues to return to their natural condition.

32. A denture bearing a tooth or teeth, made prior to the extraction appointment, so that the denture can be inserted as soon as the extraction is complete.

33. A large amount of gum shrinkage following extractions, soon leading to a poor fit.

34. a) The patient is never without teeth and therefore is able to eat and has fewer speech problems.
    b) It is easier to copy the patient's appearance
    c) Haemostasis
    d) To cover the tooth sockets.

35. a) To maintain masticatory efficiency
    b) To prevent tilting of adjacent teeth
    c) To prevent the over-eruption of unopposed teeth.

36. A cast partial upper metal denture designed as a framework rather than a full palatal coverage.

37. A metal connection joining two saddle areas of a lower partial denture.

38. a) Tissue borne, where the denture rests solely on the soft tissues
    b) Tooth borne, where all the occlusal stress is borne by the teeth
    c) Tooth/tissue - a combination of the above.

39. Retained roots or teeth. Swellings, hard or soft. White patches. Ulcers.

40. By the use of disclosing solution on the dentures.

41. They can cause perforation of the hard palate and have been known to cause cancer of the hard palate.

42. a) The ridge at the posterior border of the fitting surface of an upper denture
    b) To help produce a retention seal for the denture and to help prevent food getting under the denture.

Instrument and Material Layouts

In all cases patient notes, relevant radiographs and models must be immediately available.

Hands should be thoroughly washed at appropriate times.

All surgical instruments etc. must be sterile and laid out on sterile trays using a "no touch" technique. The tray should then be covered until used.

Bib, mouthwash, together with aspirator, spittoon or equivalent receptacle and mouth mirror should be available.

Items in brackets are less commonly required.

A conservation tray has not been listed as there is considerable variation amongst Dental Surgeons as to the instruments required.

1. Cartridge syringe. Suitable needle. Local anaesthetic cartridge, with or without vasoconstrictor as prescribed. Sterilise the end of the cartridge unless removed from a sterile pack. Warm cartridge (20-37°C).

2. Local anaesthetic tray. Upper extraction forceps - premolars. (Couplands chisel). (Gauze bite pack).

3. Local anaesthetic tray. Cheek retractor and (tongue retractor). Suitable suction tip. Aspirator. Needle holder - Ward or Kilner or some Dental Surgeons use Spencer Wells artery forceps. Toothed tissue forceps. (Tweezers). Suitable pre-sterilised suture pack or sterile half circle cutting needle and silk. Scissors. Sterile gauze squares.

4. Local anaesthetic tray. Scalpel and suitable blade. Periosteal elevator. Flap retractor e.g. Austen's. Instruments to remove bone e.g. conventional handpiece and oral surgery burs. (Mallet and chisels). Sterile water, 10ml or larger disposable syringe and needle. Elevators e.g. Warrick James, Cryers. Lower root extraction forceps. Bone trimming instruments e.g. end or side cutting bone nibblers. Suture kit.

5. Local anaesthetic tray. Scalpel and suitable blade. Formal-saline solution in labelled container with lid. Suture kit. Histopathology request form.

6. a) Rubber dam tray. Sheet of rubber. Rubber dam punch. Selection of rubber dam clamps. Rubber dam clamp forceps. Rubber dam frame or neck strap. Dental floss. Vaseline or K.Y. jelly. Saliva ejector tip and aspirator. If rubber dam is not being used; saliva ejector tip and aspirator. Cotton wool rolls.
   b) Conservation tray.
   c) Endodontic tray. Barbed broach. (Smooth broach). Set of reamers 15-140. Set of files 15-140. Paper points. Scissors. (Engine rotary paste filler). (Giromatic handpiece). (Giromatic instruments).
   d) Root dressing tray. Irrigating solution e.g. sodium hypochlorite, 1% solution. Chemical antiseptic or antibiotic paste (needle and cartridge syringe). Cotton wool pledget. Temporary filling material.

7. a) Gingival retraction cord, scissors and applicator.
   b) Suitable upper and lower impression trays.
   c) Impression for P.J.C. e.g. <u>Rubber type</u>. Impression material. Pad, spatula. Syringe. Or, <u>Ring type</u>. Copper ring. Crown scissors, tweezers. Suitable composition stick. Petroleum jelly. Gas burner, matches. Full arch locating impression e.g. alginate.
   d) Impression of opposing arch e.g. Alginate powder and measure. Mixing bowl and spatula. Adhesive. Water at 22°C and measure.
   e) Wax wafer for recording the occlusion.
   f) Shade guide.
   g) Laboratory work sheet.

8. Laboratory models plus crown or bridge. Conservation tray. (Local anaesthetic tray). Handpieces; conventional, straight and right-angled; High speed. Suitable burs to aid removal of temporary crown. Suitable burs, stones, discs etc. for any necessary trimming or polishing of crown or bridge. 3-in-1 syringe. Saliva ejector. Dental floss. Thin articulating paper. Engineer's blue. Cotton wool rolls. Suitable cement powder and liquid slab and mixing spatula.

9. Conservation tray. Saliva ejector tip and aspirator. Cotton wool. 3-in-1 syringe. Suitable lining materials, powder and liquid or pastes, slab or pad and mixing spatula. Matrix band and holder. Wedges. Alloy and mercury in amalgamator. Dappen's glass or other container for mixed amalgam. Amalgam carrier. Waste amalgam container.

10. Suitable stock or disposable impression trays, preferably perforated. Adhesive. Denture bowl. Dry tissues. Alginate powder and measure. Water at 22°C and measure. Mixing bowl and spatula. Damp tissue and sealable polythene bag for conveying impressions to the laboratory. Laboratory work sheet.

11. Laboratory models and bite blocks. Laboratory work sheet. Denture bowl. Dry tissues. Willis bite gauge or steel rule and pencil. (Fox's bite plane). (Face bow and wax wafers). Wax knife. Sheet of pink wax. Gas burner and matches. Bowl of cold water. Shade guide (mould guide).

12. Check cylinders: One full Oxygen plus one in use.
One full Nitrous Oxide plus one in use.
"FULL", "IN USE" and "EMPTY" cylinder notices available. In use cylinders turned on and giving a good flow of gas when tested. Check Emergency Oxygen working. Top up Halothane (Fluorthane) vaporizer. Check that suitable mask and anaesthetic tubes are properly connected.

13. <u>Heat</u>. Gutta percha. (Flat plastic instrument). Gas burner, matches. <u>Cold</u>. Ethyl chloride syringe. Cotton wool. College tweezers. <u>Electrical</u>. Cotton wool roll. Conducting solution. Pulp tester.

Short Essay Answers

Pathology, Microbiology and Sterilisation

1. The body's RESPONSE to INJURY (4), may be ACUTE (1) or CHRONIC (1). Redness (1), swelling, (1), warmth (1), pain (1) and loss of function (1). (11 marks).

2. a) Redness and warmth - DILATATION OF BLOOD VESSELS (1) bringing more BLOOD TO THE AREA (1)
   b) Swelling - PLASMA LEAVES THE CAPILLARIES (1) and PASSES into the TISSUES (1) (inflammatory exudate). WHITE CELLS (1) also pass through VESSEL WALLS (1)
   c) Pain - due to the EXUDATE (1) causing PRESSURE (1) on NERVE ENDINGS (1)
   d) Loss of function - caused BY PAIN (1) and by the SWELLING (1) leading to RESTRICTION (1) of movement. (12 marks).

3. a) Congenital (5). GENETIC (1) e.g. haemophilia (1). INTRA-UTERINE INFECTION (1) e.g. German measles (1). DRUGS IN PREGNANCY (1) e.g. Thalidomide (1).
   b) Acquired (5) e.g. LIVING ORGANISMS (1) - bacteria, viruses (1). DIETARY LACK (1) - rickets (1). CHEMICAL (1) - poisons (1). PHYSICAL AGENTS (1) - heat, cold, irradiation, trauma (1). (24 marks).

4. a) Natural or acquired immunity (4).
   b) Body secretions (2) - WASHING AWAY (1), and ANTI-BACTERIAL (1) action e.g. skin oils, sweat, tears, nasal secretion, saliva, etc. (2).
   c) Loss of surface cells (2).
   d) Respiratory cilia (2). (14 marks).

5. Water - at least 10 minutes (2) at constant $100^{o}C$ (2).
   a) Does not kill spores (1).
   b) Rusting (1).
   c) Steam condensation in surgery (1).

   Steam - autoclave - heating UP time (1) + $134^{o}C$ (1) for three minutes (1) + COOLING TIME (1) = cycle time of 20 minutes (1).
   a) Expense of autoclave (1).

   Hot oven - heating UP time (1) + $160^{o}C$ (1) for one hour (1) + COOLING TIME (1).
   a) Takes a LONG TIME (1).
   b) Need for extra instruments (1).
   c) Some items cannot be sterilised by this method e.g. plastics (1). (20 marks).

Anatomy and Physiology

6. Enamel forms the extremely hard (1) covering of crowns (1) of teeth. Dentine forms the bulk of tooth (1) within the enamel (1) and cementum (1). Enamel - whitish in colour (1), dentine - more yellow (1). Enamel microscopically made up of prisms (1), dentine composed of tubules (1). Enamel 96% calcium salts (1), dentine softer (1), 70% salts (1). Enamel insensitive (1), dentine sensitive (1). Enamel cannot grow once formed (1), odontoblasts line the pulpal surface of dentine and can form new dentine (1). (16 marks).

7. a) Inspiration. The rib cage EXPANDS (1), the diaphragm DESCENDS (1) as the VOLUME of the thorax increases (1), there is SUCTION pull (1) on the lung tissue so that the lungs EXPAND (1). The air PRESSURE in the lungs is now less (1) than atmospheric pressure and air FLOWS INTO the lungs (1).
   b) Expiration. The REVERSE occurs. The volume of the thorax is DECREASED (1) forcing air OUT of the lungs (1). (9 marks).

8. In the tissues (2) - capillary O_2 concentration is high (1), whilst that in the tissues is low (1), thus O_2 diffuses into the tissues (1). The reverse occurs with CO_2 (1).
In the lungs (2) - CO_2 pressure is low in the alveoli (1) and high in the blood (1), CO_2 diffuses out of the blood (1). The reverse occurs with O_2 (1). (12 marks).

9. a) Transport (2) of 1) gases (1)
2) food material (1)
3) waste products (1)
4) hormones, antibodies (1).
b) Maintenance of body water (2).
c) Regulation of body heat (2).
d) Prevention of disease (2) by circulation of
1) white cells (1)
2) antibodies (1)
3) antitoxins (1).
e) Wound plugging (2), i.e. blood clotting (1). (18 marks).

10. This is a reflex action (2). Pain stimulus (1) to the foot received by skin receptors (1). Stimulus passes along afferent nerves (1) to spinal cord (1). Reaction stimulus (1) passes along efferent nerves (1) to the leg. A motor response (1) occurs in the muscles (1) of the leg and foot, resulting in withdrawal (1) of the foot from the pin. Other impulses travel to the brain (1) which lead to controlled reactions (1) e.g. "Ouch!" (13 marks).

11. Ingestion (2) - taking in food (1). Digestion (2) - breakdown of food (1). Absorption (2) - digested food passes through lining membrane (1). Assimilation (2) - the food is used by the body cells (1). Egestion (2) - the expulsion of undigested food (1) and waste products (1). (16 marks).

Instruments, Materials and Drugs

12. To be used for SURGICAL PURPOSES ONLY (4). After use CLEANED (2) to remove blood etc. CHECK for SHARPNESS (1) and if necessary send away to be REGROUND (1). If satisfactory, lightly OIL (1) the joint, then STERILISE (2). Sterilise by DRY HEAT (2) NOT ABOVE 160°C (1) which might SPOIL THE TEMPER (1) of the metal, or by AUTOCLAVE (2) with a DRYING CYCLE (1). Moisture can cause CORROSION (1) and BLUNTNESS (1) of the blades. (20 marks).

13. a) Fixed (4) - METAL WITH RUBBER bite pads (2), or ALL RUBBER (2) e.g. HEWITT's (1) or McKESSON (1). Used to keep MOUTH OPEN (2) during GENERAL ANAESTHESIA (1); during PROLONGED CONSERVATION (1) or during SURGICAL EXTRACTION (1) under local anaesthesia.

13. b) Spring (2) - e.g. BRUNTON's (1). Used in CONSERVATION (1) and EXTRACTIONS (1) to keep the MOUTH OPEN (2). Placed in MIDLINE (1) and can be SWUNG TO NON-WORKING (1) side. (18 marks).

Note: A mouth gag is NOT a mouth prop.

14. WATER IS HEATED (1) to the TEMPERATURE RECOMMENDED (2) by the manufacturer. Suitable BOWL (1) is put out and lined with thin cloth or GAUZE (1) to prevent composition STICKING (1) to the bowl. The warm WATER is placed IN THE BOWL (1) plus the appropriate amount of COMPOSITION SLABS (1). These are allowed to SOFTEN (1), then are MOULDED (1) in the hands, replaced in the water to RESOFTEN, then REMOULDED (1). The composition should then be EVENLY SOFT (1) and should be left in the water prior to loading the impression tray. In some surgeries an electrically heated warm water bath will be used to keep the composition ready for use all the time. This composition needs moulding to ensure even softness. (12 marks).

15. a) It should not affect the health of the patient (2) or the oral tissues (2).
b) It should be able to withstand acid foods (1) etc.
c) It should not react with other materials (2) in the oral environment to produce galvanic (1) or other unwanted effects (1).
d) It should expand and contract (2) with temperature changes (1) in a similar manner to the tooth tissues (1).
e) It should be able to withstand high masticatory forces (2).
f) It should have a pleasing appearance (1).
g) It should have sufficient working time (1) and set within a reasonable period of time (1).
h) It should have minimum corrosion (1). (19 marks).

16. All containers must be PROPERLY LABELLED (4). Labels should carry information on NAME OF CONTENTS (2), STRENGTH OF CONTENTS (2), DATE OF PURCHASE and/or EXPIRY (1) to reduce out of date stock being used. Contents of UNLABELLED CONTAINERS should be DISCARDED (2). Stock should be kept TIDY (1), this will reduce OVERSTOCKING (1). All drugs must be kept in a SAFE PLACE (1), preferably a lockable cupboard (1). Storage should be in COOL DRY (1) conditions unless the manufacturer ADVISES OTHERWISE (1). Drugs of ADDICTION (2) and drugs acting on the CENTRAL NERVOUS system (2) must be kept in a LOCKED CUPBOARD (2). Maintain a record of PURCHASE (1) and USE (1) of drugs. This will also be useful in STOCK CONTROL (1). All poisons should be clearly labelled POISON (2). (28 marks).

17. a) Orally (2) e.g. analgesic tablets or capsules (1).
    b) Injection (2) e.g. local anaesthetic solution, intravenous sedation or anaesthesia, intra-muscular antibiotics (1).
    c) Topically (2) via mucous membrane e.g. anaesthetic ointment, (1).
    d) Inhalation (2) e.g. nitrous oxide, Halothane, decongestants for sinusitis (1). (12 marks).

Dental Disease

18. Clinical
    a) LABIAL CARIES (2) of deciduous teeth where COMFORTERS (1) containing CONCENTRATED SYRUPS (1) and fruit juices have been used a lot.
    b) SUDDEN INCREASE (2) in number of NEW CAVITIES (1) in OLDER PATIENTS (2) if the amount of SWEET EATING (1) is greatly increased.

    Epidemiological
    a) LACK OF CARIES in PRIMITIVE PEOPLES (2) until civilisation reaches them, and they eat a "modern" diet (1).
    b) FALL OF CARIES (2) rate during Second World War when there was SUGAR RATIONING (1).

    Experimental
    VIPEHOLME STUDY (2). This showed the greatest INCREASE (2) in caries with frequent BETWEEN MEALS (1) consumption of SUGAR (1) in STICKY form. This effect was REVERSED (2) when patients RETURNED (1) to a basic diet UNSUPPLEMENTED (1) by sugar. (26 marks).

19. NONE BETWEEN (3) meals. A FEW after ONE MEAL (3) on SOME DAYS. CLEAN TEETH (3) afterwards or RINSE MOUTH (1). Sticky SWEETS (2) should be kept to a minimum. (12 marks).

20. More PLAQUE (2), more CALCULUS (2), LOSS OF ALVEOLAR bone (2), LOOSENING OF TOOTH (2), eventual LOSS OF the tooth (2). (10 marks).

21. Supragingival (2)
    a) Teeth involved mainly lower incisors and upper molars (2).
    b) Colour - yellowish (1).
    c) Site - above gum (1).
    d) Chalky consistency - not too difficult to remove (1).

    Subgingival (2)
    a) Any teeth can be involved (2).
    b) Colour - black (1).
    c) Site - below gum (1).
    d) Hard and tenacious (1). (14 marks).

22. This answer must relate to the process of acute inflammation. The pulp is INFECTED (2) and INFLAMED (2) there is INCREASED BLOOD SUPPLY (2) to the area and formation of INFLAMMATORY EXUDATE (2). There CANNOT (1) be any SWELLING within a hard substance, therefore PRESSURE INCREASES (2), STIMULATING NERVE ENDINGS (1) and causing severe pain. If this PRESSURE IS RELIEVED (2) i.e. into the MOUTH (1) or into the SOFTER TISSUES (1) in the periapical area, there will be RELIEF OF PAIN (2). (18 marks).

23. a) Naturally (2) by tooth substance CRUMBLING away (1) to produce a SELF-cleansing surface (1).
    b) Artificially (2) by a Dental Surgeon who either GRINDS AWAY (1) tooth substance to produce a SELF-cleansing area (1) or by CAVITY preparation (2) and FILLING (2). (12 marks).

24. a) Decalcification (2). ACIDS (1) are produced by the action of BACTERIA on CARBOHYDRATES (1). These ACIDS (1) break down CALCIUM SALTS (1) in the tooth substance.
    b) Proteolysis (2). Certain BACTERIA (1), present in the mouth, DIGEST (1) the ORGANIC content (1) of the tooth. (11 marks).

25. So that MINIMAL PLAQUE (2) is left on the teeth at night. Whilst we are asleep there are MINIMAL MOVEMENTS OF THE TONGUE (2) and very LITTLE SALIVA (2) is produced. Plaque therefore remains UNDISTURBED (2) and leads to prolonged ATTACK (2) on dental tissues. (10 marks).

Restorative Dentistry

26. a) Saliva ejector (1) and cotton wool rolls (1) - to keep the cavity dry (1).
    b) Cavity oil or grease - to aid the removal of the impression (1).
    c) Blue inlay wax (1) the impression material (1).
    d) Gas or spirit burner (1) to soften the inlay wax (1).
    e) Wax carving instruments (1) e.g. the Ward wax carver - to carve the wax before its removal from the cavity (1).
    f) Metal sprue (1) to remove the impression from the cavity (1), for transport to the laboratory.
    g) Container (1) in which to transport the impression to the laboratory (1). (14 marks).

27. a) By a COMPLETE LAY-OUT (2) of:- patients' RECORDS (1) including RADIOGRAPHS (1), necessary INSTRUMENTS (1) and MATERIALS (1).
b) By ANTICIPATION (2) in the passing of INSTRUMENTS (1) and having MATERIALS (1) ready for use.
c) By TAKING OVER (2) some actions from the Dental Surgeon e.g. SHORTENING (1) a paper point, and WETTING (1) it in root canal antiseptic. (14 marks).

28. a) By having necessary instruments (2) and materials (2) available but not on display (1).
b) Making sure the patient is seen on time (2).
c) If opportune, by showing the child how the equipment works (1).
d) Playing a supporting role to the Dental Surgeon (1).
e) By stressing to the child the importance of oral hygiene (1). (10 marks).

29. a) Not to spill mercury (1).
b) Keep mercury and waste amalgam in sealed containers (2).
c) Not to wear open-toed shoes (1).
d) Not to handle mercury or mixed amalgam (2).
e) Make sure room is well-ventilated (1).
f) Possibly keep the amalgamator in an enclosed container (1).
g) Use a rubber sheet or finger stall to cover the dental napkin when squeezing out excess mercury (2).
h) Wash hands after using amalgam (1). (11 marks).

30. a) Inform the Dental Surgeon (2).
b) Wearing rubber gloves and face mask (4).
   1) Carefully collect obvious mercury into a suitable vessel (2).
   2) To prevent globules running, spread dry sand (2) over the area and then sweep (2) the area taking special care to empty any surface cracks (2).
c) All the spilt mercury should be stored in a closed container under water (2). (16 marks).

Anaesthesia, First Aid and Minor Oral Surgery

31. a) Relatively easy to administer (3).
b) Simpler equipment (1).
c) Can be used on most patients some of whom might be unfit for general anaesthesia (3).
d) Initial control of haemorrhage in surgical cases (2) if solution containing vasoconstrictor used adjacent to site of surgery.
e) Patient co-operation throughout procedures (2).
f) No time constraints (1).
g) Less risk to the patient (2). (14 marks).

32. The anaesthetic drug WORKS ON THE BRAIN (3) but is ADMINISTERED AT SOME REMOTE POINT (3) e.g. LUNGS (1) or VEIN (1) in the hand. The drug also induces a state of unconsciousness (3). (11 marks).

33. a) ANTICIPATION OF NEEDS (2) of the Surgeon or the Anaesthetist, depending upon whom she is assisting.
    b) PASSING INSTRUMENTS (2) etc.
    c) Keeping operating FIELD CLEAR (2) by careful RETRACTION (1) and good SUCTION (1).
    d) Assisting in MONITORING (2) of the patient's respiration and pulse.
    e) Acting as CHAPERONE (2).
    f) Forming part of the SURGERY TEAM (1). (13 marks).

34. a) Supporting the patient's head to MAINTAIN THE AIRWAY (3) and to PREVENT the patient INJURING (3) himself.
    b) MONITOR respiration (2) and pulse (2).
    c) Use SUCTION (1) to remove BLOOD (1) and SALIVA (1) from the mouth if necessary.
    d) Ensure that, if the patient should vomit, NONE IS INHALED (3). (16 marks).

35. a) The patient should be laid on his/her back (2) on a firm surface (2).
    b) Any possible airway obstruction (2) should be removed, e.g. foreign body (1) such as denture, or constriction such as tight collar (1).
    c) Extend the patient's neck and insert a neck roll (3). Hold the jaw forward (1) (to prevent the tongue obstructing the airway) (1).
    d) Pinch the nostrils (2).
    e) Place your mouth over the patient's mouth (2) ensuring a seal (1).
    f) Blow into the patient's mouth (1) checking that the chest rises (2). If no chest movement find cause of obstruction (2).
    g) Maintain a rate of at least ten breaths per minute (1). (24 marks).

In the surgery: insert oral airway (2), cover the nose and mouth with close fitting (1) face mask (2) connected to the oxygen supply (2). Inflate lungs with oxygen (2) by squeezing the respiratory bag (2). In all cases help should be summoned (1) and an attempt made to diagnose the cause of the condition (1). (13 marks).

36. a) The patient should be laid on the floor (2); this is an easier working position (1). Kneel beside the patient (1).
b) The heels of the hands (1) are placed on top of each other (1) over the lower half (1) of the patient's sternum (1).
c) The sternum should be depressed about one and a half inches (1) by applying your full weight. Repeat this once per second (1).
d) Depressing the sternum will squeeze the heart against the spine (2) forcing blood into the circulatory system (2). (14 marks).

37. a) Lay the patient flat (1) or in the tonsillar position (2). (Putting the head between the knees may compress the inferior vena cava, and in fact reduce the blood flow from the legs). Ideally the legs should be raised above the level of the heart and brain (1) to ensure the blood supply to the brain (1).
b) Remove any possible airway obstruction (2) e.g. denture, tight collar.
c) If necessary administer oxygen (1).
d) As the patient recovers, reassure (1), but keep him flat (1).
e) As the patient's colour returns, raise him slowly (1), but lower again if signs of fainting again, are seen (1).
f) Give the patient a glucose drink (1) to raise the blood sugar level which is sometimes low in patients who faint. (13 marks).

38. Before (2)
a) Get out the patient's NOTES (1) and RADIOGRAPHS (1).
b) STERILISE (2) all the necessary INSTRUMENTS (1), WASH HANDS (1), LAY INSTRUMENTS OUT ON A TRAY (1) using 'NON TOUCH TECHNIQUES' (2). Cover tray with STERILE COVER (1).
c) Get the CORRECT PATIENT ready and comfortably SEATED in the chair (1).

During (2)
a) After SCRUBBING HANDS (1) be prepared to RETRACT TISSUES (1), use SUCTION (1) and PASS INSTRUMENTS (1) as required. ANTICIPATE (2) Surgeon's requirements.
b) MONITOR (2) and if necessary, REASSURE (1) the patient.

After (2)
a) Make sure the patient is CLEANED UP (1) and FIT ENOUGH (2) to leave the surgery.
b) Make sure the patient understands all POST-OPERATIVE INSTRUCTIONS (2).
c) CLEAN (1) and STERILISE (2) all the instruments.
d) Clean all the WORKING SURFACES (1) and attend to the SUCKER (1). (36 marks).

Multiple Choice Answers

General

1. d)	2. a)	3. a)	4. d)
5. c)	6. a)	7. e)	8. d)
9. b)	10. d)	11. d)	12. a)
13. d)	14. d)	15. b)	16. c)
17. c)	18. b)		

Oral Anatomy

19. c)	20. b)	21. c)	22. c)
23. a)	24. e)	25. a)	26. c)
27. e)	28. e)	29. d)	30. 1) d) 2) h) 3) g) 4) b) 5) e)
31. 1) h) 2) j) 3) c) 4) f) 5) d)	32. 1) i) 2) c) 3) a) d) 4) b) e) f) h) j)		33. c)
34. b)	35. c)	36. d)	37. b) d)
38. e)	39. e)	40. b)	41. b)
42. c)	43. a)	44. a)	45. e)
46. e)	47. e)		

Microbiology

48. c) d)	49. a)	50. a) or c)	51. d)
52. b) e)	53. a)	54. d)	55. a) b)
56. a) 6) b) 1) c) 7) d) 3)			

Materials

57. c)	58. c)	59. c)	60. a)
61. a)	62. e)	63. e)	64. c)
65. a) b)	66. c) e)	67. b)	68. e)
69. b)	70. a) d)		

Prosthetics

71. d)	72. a) c) d)	73. a) d)	74. b)
75. a) b)	76. e)	77. c) d)	78. b)
79. b)	80. c)	81. c)	82. c) e)
83. b)	84. a) e)	85. e)	86. c)
87. a) b) c)	88. b)	89. e)	
90. a) c) e)			

Radiography

91. c)	92. c)	93. d) e)	94. a) d)
95. a) c)	96. c)	97. a)	
98. a) b) c)	99. a)	100. a) b)	101. a)
102. a) b)	103. b)	104. a) d)	
105. a) b) c)	106. c) d)	107. d)	108. b)
109. d)	110. a) 6) b) 3) c) 5)	111. a) 1) 9) 5) b) 8) 4) c) 7) 3)	

Anaesthesia

112. a) d)	113. 1) a) 2) b) 3) f)	114. b)	115. a)
116. a) e)	117. b) c)	118. d)	119. a) d)
120. b)	121. e)	122. d)	123. b) c)
124. b)	125. 1) b) 2) a) 3) b) 4) c) or b) 5) b) 6) a) or b)		126. b)
127. 1) c) 2) f) 3) b) 4) b) f) 5) d)	128. a)	129. c)	130. d)
131. a)	132. a)	133. d)	134. e)
135. b)	136. c)		

Caries

137. a)	138. e)	139. d)	140. b)
141. a)	142. a) d)	143. e)	144. c)
145. a) c)	146. c)	147. d)	148. c) e)
149. b)	150. e)	151. d)	

Children's Dentistry

152. b)	153. c)	154. b)	155. a)
156. e)	157. d) e)	158. a)	159. b)
160. a) d)	161. b)	162. d)	163. b) c)
164. b)	165. a)	166. b)	167. a)
168. b)	169. b)	170. c) e)	171. a)
172. a)	173. a) b) c) d)		174. b)
175. e)	176. a)		

Conservation

177. d)	178. b) c)	179. c)	180. a)
181. a)	182. a) b)	183. d)	
184. b) c) d)	185. a) d)	186. b) c)	187. e) b)
188. b) c)	189. a) b) e)	190. 1) d) 2) b) 3) f) 4) a)	
191. b) d) e)	192. a) c) d)	193. c)	194. a)
195. b) d)	196. a)	197. e)	198. b)
199. a) e)	200. e)	201. a) c)	
202. b) i) e) d) f)		203. b) d) e) f) h)	
204. b)	205. b) e)	206. a)	
207. a) d) b)	208. b) d)	209. d)	210. b)